30-MINUTE DIETWALK®
FOR WOMEN

LOSE 12 LBS., SHAPE UP, & LOOK YOUNGER IN 2 WEEKS

FRED A. STUTMAN, M.D.

MEDICAL MANOR BOOKS
PHILADELPHIA, PA

30-Minute Dietwalk® For Women

Publisher's Cataloging-in-Publication

Names: Stutman, Fred A., author.

Title: 30-minute dietwalk for women : Lose 12 Lbs., Shape Up, & Look Younger in 2 Weeks / Fred A. Stutman, M.D.

Other titles: Thirty-minute dietwalk for women

Description: First edition. | Philadelphia, PA : Medical Manor Books, [2017] | Includes bibliographical references and index.

Identifiers: ISBN: 978-0-934232-48-7 (paperback) | 978-0-934232-49-4 (ebook) | LCCN: 2015905087

Subjects: LCSH: Women--Health and hygiene. | Reducing exercises. | Reducing diets. | Women-- Nutrition. | Physical fitness for women. | Fitness walking. | BISAC: HEALTH & FITNESS / General. | HEALTH & FITNESS / Aerobics. | HEALTH & FITNESS / Diet & Nutrition / Weight Loss. | HEALTH & FITNESS / Diet & Nutrition / Nutrition. | HEALTH & FITNESS / Diet & Nutrition / Diets. | HEALTH & FITNESS / Diet & Nutrition / General.

Classification: LCC: RA778 .S887 2017 | DDC: 613.7/045--dc23

First Edition 2017
Manufactured in the United States of America

OTHER BOOKS BY THE AUTHOR:

Walk, Don't Run. Philadelphia: Medical Manor Press, 1979.

The Doctor's Walking Book. New York: Ballantine Books, 1980.

The Doctor's Walking Diet. Philadelphia: Medical Manor Books, 1982.

DietWalk: The Doctor's Fast 3-Day SuperDiet. Philadelphia: Medical Manor Books, 1983. Pocket Books® Edition, Simon & Schuster, New York, 1987.

Walk, Don't Die. Philadelphia: Medical Manor Books, 1986. Bart Books Edition: New York, 1988.

Walk To Win: The Easy 4-Day Diet & Fitness Plan. Philadelphia: Medical Manor Books, 1990.

Diet-Step: 20/20-For Women Only. Philadelphia: Medical Manor Books, 2001.

Diet-Step: For Seniors. Philadelphia: Medical Manor Books, 2003.

100 Best Weight-Loss Tips. Philadelphia: Medical Manor Books, 2005.

100 Weight-Loss Tips That Really Work. New York: McGraw Hill Books, 2007.

Dr. Walk's Power Diet-Step. Philadelphia: Medical Manor Books, 2009.

The Case of the Unwanted Pounds. Philadelphia: Medical Manor Books, 2011.

Philly's Fit-Step Walking Diet. Philadelphia: Medical Manor Books, 2014.

Medical Manor Books are available at special quantity discounts for sales promotions, premiums, fund raising or educational use. Book excerpts can also be created to fit special needs.

For details write the
Special Markets Dept. of Medical Manor Books
3501 Newberry Road, Philadelphia, PA 19154

Phone: 800-DIETING (343-8464)
E-mail: info@medicalmanorbooks.com
Website: www.medicalmanorbooks.com

To Suzanne

ACKNOWLEDGMENTS

EDITOR: Suzanne Stutman, Ph.D.

PERMISSIONS: The American Academy of Family Practice; J & J Snack Foods, Inc.; The Physicians' Health Bulletin; Dr. Walk's Diet & Fitness Newsletter

COVER DESIGN: Alex Shin

TEXT DESIGN: Erin Howarth

PUBLISHER: Medical Manor Books, Philadelphia, PA

DIETWALK® is the registered trademark of Dr. Stutman's Quick Weight-Loss & Body-Shaping Plan.

DR. WALK® is the registered trademark of Dr. Stutman's Diet & Fitness Newsletter.

DIET-STEP® is the registered trademark of Dr. Stutman's Weight-Loss Program.

FIT-STEP® is the registered trademark of Dr. Stutman's Fitness Walking Program.

CONTENTS

9: LOOK YOUNGER & LIVE LONGER! 153

10: FAT & FIBER COUNTER 173

SUBJECT INDEX 215

AUTHOR'S CAUTION

IT IS ESSENTIAL THAT YOU CONSULT YOUR OWN PHYSICIAN BEFORE BEGINNING THE 30-MINUTE DIETWALK PLAN FOR WOMEN.

-Fred A. Stutman, M.D.

Introduction

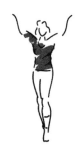

Dietwalk Plan for Women

If you really want to lose six pounds every week and become physically fit in just 14 days, all you have to do is follow the easy DietWalk Plan for Women.

Nobody really wants to follow a diet or an exercise program. They are nothing more than a pain in the butt. Dieting in general involves too much thought, preparation, and effort. Whether you are following the artery clogging, high fat, low carbohydrate diets, or trying another gimmick diet, you are actually not getting the essential nutrients that your body needs. Not to mention the good tasting foods that you can't have on any of these restrictive, fad diets.

And as far as exercise is concerned, there is no doubt in anyone's mind that exercise is really a bore and most exercises usually are just too strenuous and time consuming. Jump up, lift that, squat here, run there, or any one of a dozen useless body gyrations that leave us huffing and puffing. At most gyms, you have to use a variety of machines in order to exercise each group of muscles in your body. Then you start thinking, "Did I exercise my triceps or was it my biceps?" "Was I already on that machine, or was that machine in a different row?" "All of these machines look the same and now I have to start all over again since I don't know where I began."

How about the stair climber or the elliptical machine? Aren't they supposed to be good for you? Well in moderation yes, but have you ever watched those enthusiastic, compulsive people exercising on these machines. They go faster and faster and the veins bulge in their necks and they're drenched in perspiration, and yet they never stop. Is this fun? Can this be good for you? I think not! Studies have repeatedly shown that strenuous exercises, rather than being beneficial, are actually detrimental to our health. Strenuous exercises and lifting heavy weights can actually raise our blood pressures and make us more susceptible to irregular heart rhythms. And of course, there is all of the muscle and joint and ligament injuries that all of these over enthusiastic exercisers sustain over and over again. Won't they ever learn? I think not. People have been brainwashed into thinking that if an exercise is not painful or strenuous, then it can't be good for you. This is the so-called **"no-pain no-gain myth."** Nothing could be further from the truth. Medical studies have repeatedly shown that moderate exercise is far more beneficial and less detrimental to our health than those back-breaking, gut-wrenching, limb-straining types of exercises.

You don't really have to join a gym or a fitness club to exercise. You don't have to engage in lung-straining, muscle-wrenching, or heart-racing exercises in order to lose weight and get fit. And you do not have to subject your body to all of the torturous exercises that the so-called fitness gurus have brainwashed everyone into believing are essential for weight loss and fitness. So, what do we do? Just sit there! Not really! The answer is simple. All you have to do is follow the **DietWalk Plan for Women**, which consists of an easy-to-follow diet and exercise plan that will allow you **to lose six pounds every week** and **in just 14 days, your body will be fit, trim, firm and energized.**

Sound easy? It is! And believe me, it works without any of the dangers or hazards involved in strenuous exercises or by using heavy weights for strength training and muscle building. **You'll see the following results in just 14 days on the DietWalk Plan for Women:**

- You can lose up to 12 lbs. in only 2 weeks
- Stronger muscles and bones
- Better muscle sculpting and definition
- Improved health and cardiovascular fitness
- Considerably more energy every day
- Feeling good about yourself
- The ability to cope better with stress and tension
- Feeling of well-being and improved self-image
- Being able to relax and cope easily with daily problems
- Feeling at peace with yourself and with others.

The **DietWalk Plan for Women** has the following essential key points:

- Low-fat and low refined carbohydrate (bad carbs) foods.
- High fiber complex good carbohydrate foods.
- Moderate lean protein foods.
- Non-fat dairy calcium and protein containing products.
- Walking 30 minutes six days per week.
- Walk for 30 minutes, three days per week, using hand-held weights for strength training and calorie burning.

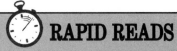 **RAPID READS**

If you're in a rush to lose weight, turn to the back of every chapter to read the most important points, then go back when you have time to read more detailed explanations.

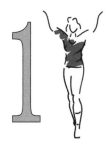

THE DIETWALK MYSTERY

This diet and fitness program was designed especially for women who have tried various quick weight-loss fad diets and who, unfortunately, seem to have unwanted pounds that actually never come off. Even more frustrating is the fact that once they have finished with their diets, they usually gain back more weight than they lost before they started the diet. This is called "rebound weight-gain," which is all too common with most if not all fad diets. Many women also have been told that strenuous exercises will help them to lose weight and become physically fit, only to find that these types of exercises will not cause permanent weight loss or lasting fitness, and may in fact do more harm than good.

The easy steps presented in The DIETWALK Plan solve the mystery of how to lose weight quickly and permanently and how to achieve maximum cardiovascular fitness. In addition, this plan shows you how to prevent the degenerative diseases of aging including heart attacks, hypertension, strokes, and certain forms of cancer. This unique diet and fitness program reveals the hazards of unhealthy fad diets and strenuous exercises, and illuminates the benefits of a truly healthy permanent weight-loss diet plan, and a safe and effective fitness plan. The DIETWALK Plan shows you how to lose weight, get fit, and look younger.

MODERN-DAY DIET CHARLATANS

How do people lose weight on all of those popular low-carbohydrate, high-fat diets? For example, they say you can have bacon and eggs for breakfast, hot dogs for lunch, and a juicy steak for dinner. Sounds tempting, doesn't it? They also tell you that you can't have any, or at the very least, limited amounts of carbohydrates with each meal. For instance: no vegetables, fruits, cereals, breads, potatoes, pasta, or any whole-grain nutritious foods or desserts. Sounds unappetizing and unhealthy, doesn't it? It certainly is! And yet, over 75% of the commercially available so-called diet plans work on this abnormal metabolic process principle.

The simple fact is that you do lose weight, initially, on these very low carbohydrate, high fat, high protein diets. However, most of the initial weight loss is water weight loss, due to a metabolic process called *ketosis*, which in fact is a condition found in unhealthy patients (for example, those with diabetes and kidney disease), not in healthy people. Once the body gets rid of the water, it starts burning fat, which is left over—which, in itself, is a good thing; however, the downside is that this abnormal process of ketosis also begins to burn the body's protein (muscle tissue), which is very dangerous. By attempting to burn protein as a source of fuel for energy, the body is actually breaking down one of its most important elements in the body, protein, which is used to sustain life (building and repairing the body's tissues, cells and organs). The fact that a substance called ketones appears in your urine (a byproduct of this abnormal process called *ketosis*), shows you clear evidence that your body is breaking down its muscle tissue. This is one of the reasons that fatigue and general weakness have been reported as early side effects of this completely unhealthy diet. Also, kidney and liver damage may result if too much of the body's protein is broken down from these unhealthy diets. And to make matters worse, these diets are deficient in vitamins, minerals, and essential nutrients.

These rapid weight loss programs (low-carbohydrate, high-fat, and high-protein diets) also have the added downside of what's called "rebound weight gain." This occurs after the initial weight loss, which results from fat and protein breakdown used for energy production (fuel). The body's carbohydrate stores then become depleted because of the very low intake of carbohydrates in these diets, and thus, there is limited availability of carbohydrate to be burned as a fuel. Unfortunately, these low stores of carbohydrates are designed to be the very first type of calories to be burned as fuel in our normal metabolism.

Once your body becomes aware that it is carbohydrate depleted by exhibiting the symptoms of fatigue, malaise, muscle cramps, and decreased urine output, which occurs after the initial water loss, then your brain's control center receives stress (SOS) signals from all of the body's cells suffering from carbohydrate depletion. Once your brain's central control center receives this flood of distress messages, it immediately realizes it needs a cheaper source of fuel (refined carbohydrate and sugar) to prevent brain damage from the lack of glucose that the brain needs in order to function. Just when you're feeling exhausted and done in by this enemy low-carb diet, your hunger center sets you off on a carbohydrate binge, to counteract this lethargy you've been feeling for weeks or months. And then your body explodes into its former overweight self, hence the term "rebound weight gain." Eventually, your sweet tooth gets satisfied, and then you resume your unhealthy diet of excess fat and low carbohydrates. Not a pretty picture, is it?

DIETWALK'S METABOLISM MYSTERY

I. HOW YOUR BODY BURNS CALORIES (FUEL)

A. BASAL METABOLIC RATE: Just eating food burns calories! Sounds too good to be true, but it actually is a fact. Your body burns up a certain number of calories from the foods that you eat (carbohydrates, fat, and protein) and turns part of it into fuel that you need to function every day. Protein, carbohydrate, and fat each burn a different number of calories in this conversion process. If your body realizes there are not enough calories in your diet, it switches to a slower metabolic rate in an attempt to protect you from starvation, as in times of famine—it's a natural physiologic reaction.

Unfortunately, obese people stay in the slow metabolic rate mode because they usually go on and off diets frequently; consequently, it becomes difficult for them to lose weight. The metabolic rate stays in the slow mode because the body never knows when it will get enough food to sustain life. Then, at times when there are excess calories in your diet, weight is easily gained.

B. EXERCISE: The most important way to burn calories is by exercise. This certainly is a more efficient method of losing weight than by just relying on your body to burn calories by the sedentary process of just eating food.

1. Fast, quick, physical exercise such as jogging, running, tennis, basketball, racquetball, strenuous aerobic exercises, and race walking, burns primarily carbohydrate stores in the production of energy.

2. Slow, repetitious physical activity such as walking and swimming burns primarily fat stored in the body, which is the best type of exercise for sustained weight loss.

C. FOODS THAT WE EAT: In general, we burn almost all of the protein and carbohydrates that we eat every day. We store the remaining carbohydrates in our muscles and liver in the form of a chemical compound called *glycogen*. This glycogen is used for the future production of energy. The difference between the energy supplied by protein and carbohydrate in our diets and our total energy requirements each day has to come from burning fats.

Weight gain actually occurs from taking in more calories in the form of dietary fats than were burned off as fuel for energy. On a low-fat diet, calories are removed from storage in fat cells and are added to the fuel mixture of protein and carbohydrate for the production of energy. This results in steady, permanent weight loss, unlike the temporary water weight loss of low-carbohydrate, high-protein diets. It's simple—*less fat taken in results in more storage fat being burned as fuel,* resulting in more fat lost from your body. More fat taken in results in more fat being stored, and less fat being burned, and lumpy, unsightly fat cells remaining!

II. HOW YOUR BODY CHANGES FOOD INTO ENERGY

A. PROTEIN in our diet is not a significant factor in weight regulation. Almost all of the energy contained in the protein that you eat is burned as fuel for the body's metabolic process of functioning (living). Hardly any of the calories contained in dietary protein is converted into fat storage. Only 75% of the energy contained in protein can be used for your metabolic processes such as repairing the body cells, because it takes almost 25% of the energy in protein just to change it into a form that our body can use to build and repair the body's cells, tissues, and organs.

B. FAT, on the other hand, is easily converted into energy. Almost 95% of the dietary fat calories can be stored in fat cells when you take in excess calories of fat in your diet. In other words—*it is the fat in your diet that makes you fat!* It is not necessarily the number of calories in your diet that makes you fat, it is the number of fat calories that makes you fat.

C. CARBOHYDRATES: Before we can discuss a healthy weight loss program, we have to talk briefly about carbohydrates. Carbohydrates are the body's natural source of fuel to produce energy. One of the most important basic metabolic functions of the body is to use almost all of the carbohydrate calories you eat, as a source of fuel for energy production.

The leftover carbohydrate calories not immediately used for fuel to produce energy are stored in your liver and your muscles as glycogen, which is stored as a ready source of fuel whenever the body needs it. It is readily available and can be retrieved from the liver and muscles into the bloodstream easily, where it is quickly converted to a substance called glucose (sugar), where it then becomes available to burn as a fuel for energy production. Only 5 to 10% of the carbohydrate that you eat is converted as storage into fat cells. That amounts to almost 90% being available for immediate or reserve fuel for energy production, without hardly any of the carbohydrate that you eat being converted into fat. To put it simply—*complex carbohydrates in your diet will not make you fat!*

Your body expends 2½ times more energy converting dietary carbohydrate calories from your intestines into your bloodstream for immediate energy use than it takes to convert fat into a source of fuel for energy production. This means that almost all of the excess fat calories that you eat are stored in fat cells, and end up staying there indefinitely. In other words, a *high complex carbohydrate, low-fat diet* causes your body to work harder after each meal burning calories for energy, compared to a high-fat, low-carbohydrate diet. This means that your basal metabolic rate (the rate at which your body operates all of its functions) is considerably higher on the high-carbohydrate, low-fat diet. This higher basal metabolic rate results in an additional burning of approximately 250 calories daily by the simple *thermic effect* of converting carbohydrates into energy.

III. How Your Body Stores Fuel

A. FAT: Fat is stored in fat cells (adipose tissue) in a ratio of four parts fat and one part water. Since there are *nine calories in each gram of fat*, it means that one pound of fat contains 3500 calories! It therefore takes a deficit of 3500 calories to lose just one pound of fat.

Fat, unfortunately, can be stored in unlimited quantities. Normal weight individuals have almost 100,000 calories stored in fat cells. By increasing fat in the diet, combined with a sedentary life style, it is quite easy to add another 50,000 to 100,000 calories in fat stores, increasing your weight 15 to 30 pounds every year. The only way to lose even one pound of body weight is to burn approximately 3500 calories. This can only be accomplished by cutting back on the amount of fat in the diet, and by increasing physical activity. Nothing else works! One of my favorite sayings to my patients when they ask me how to lose weight is: *"The only way you can lose weight is to eat less and walk more, or you can walk more and eat less!"*

B. CARBOHYDRATES: Carbohydrates that we eat are changed into a type of sugar (glucose in the bloodstream) to be used as an immediate source of fuel for the production of energy. Since only a small amount of the carbohydrates we eat is changed into immediate fuel sources, the majority of the carbohydrates consumed are changed into glycogen for storage in the liver and muscles. There are only 4 calories in each gram of carbohydrate (not 9 calories as in fat).

Glycogen is stored in the liver and muscles in a ratio of one part glycogen to four parts water (just the opposite of fat storage which is four parts fat to one part water). The liver's capacity to store glycogen is limited to approximately 500 calories and the muscles can store about 1500 calories. Muscle tissue, however, can store extra calories when you exercise so that your muscles burn energy more efficiently. When you increase your glycogen stores by 500 calories, you will gain a pound of body weight and when you decrease your glycogen stores by 500 calories, you will lose a pound of body weight. This weight, as you can see from the above ratio of glycogen to water, is mostly water weight.

THE DIETWALK PLAN

Remember, you live in your body and you do not have to make drastic changes in order to feel good about yourself. The DietWalk Plan will enable you to lose as much weight as you want in order to feel comfortable with your body. You will also develop maximum cardiovascular fitness, a firm, toned body and boundless energy on this wonderful new program. This plan was developed for my patients, who like most of you, were tired of the endless, short-lived fad diets and the myriad of strenuous exercise programs that are completely unrealistic.

The problem with most diet and exercise programs is that they are too complicated. There are too many tables to consult, too many diet meal plans to prepare and too many strenuous exercises to do. Most of these plans don't realize that everyone has a life to lead that is packed full of a hundred things to do each week. People don't really have the time to follow any type of complicated or time-consuming diet or weight-loss plans. The beauty of the DIETWALK Plan is that it is designed especially for women who have limited amounts of time for diet and exercise, but who would like a simple, easy, effective weight-loss plan that doesn't interfere with the rest of their lives. It's that simple! It's easy and effective, it doesn't take a lot of your valuable time, and it actually works!

I originally developed this program for my patients, who wanted a diet and exercise plan that doesn't interfere with day-to-day living. You'll be delighted at how easy the program is, and how well it works. The DietWalk Plan is easy to follow and will help you to lose weight and keep fit and healthy. There are no complicated diet plans to follow, no diet shakes to consume or weight-loss clinics to join. This is a truly simple, easy to follow, effective weight-loss program with a minimum of time and effort on your part.

Different people respond very differently to diet and fitness programs. The secret of The DietWalk Plan is that it takes all of that into consideration in the formulation of the plan. This program is designed for people of all ages and all types of body builds. It doesn't matter whether you're slightly overweight or obese, short or tall, athletic or unconditioned, young or old, muscular or flabby—this is the perfect weight-loss plan for you. This weight-loss program is not only geared towards your individual body build, but also towards your metabolic rate and your body's chemical composition. This plan will also boost your energy level and increase your metabolism as you burn off unwanted fat calories, and easily lose those unwanted pounds. You can actually *lose up to 12 pounds in only 2 weeks*. As Benjamin Franklin once said, *"One should eat to live, not live to eat."*

THE DIETWALK STEPS

STEP 1: DIETWALK® 30/30 PLAN

The 1st step consists of a diet of no more than *30 grams of total fat* and no less than *30 grams of fiber* each day. The quick weight-loss formula combines foods that are low in saturated fats and high in heart-healthy monounsaturated fats. Also, the diet limits refined, bad carbohydrates and substitutes healthy complex good carbohydrates, consisting of fruits, vegetables, and whole-grain products. The Diet-Step Plan lets you lose weight at your own pace without complicated diet plans, counting calories, fad diets, or starvation techniques. The plan is easy-to-follow and quite effective for losing weight quickly and maintaining the weight that you've lost.

1. *Decrease the amount of saturated fats in your diet* which includes fatty meats, fatty fowl like duck and dark meat of chicken and turkey; whole dairy products including butter, margarine, and hydrogenated or partially hydrogenated oils (corn, palm, safflower and other vegetable oils). These oils are also present in the form of trans-fats contained in prepared, packaged, and processed foods like chips, cookies, crackers, cake mixes, frozen dinners, margarine, vegetable spreads, and any and all products that contain trans fats. Limit your total fat intake to no more than 30 grams daily for good health and weight loss. By limiting your total fat intake, you will automatically limit your intake of unhealthy saturated fats.

2. *Increase the amounts of heart-healthy monounsaturated fats with omega-3 fatty acids,* such as olive oil, canola oils and peanut oils, nuts and seeds, all types of beans and legumes, avocados, fish and flax seeds. Use non-fat or 1% milk, yogurt and cheeses and soy protein products. Also, include the new heart healthy vegetable spreads, e.g. Promise®, Benecol®, Smart Balance®, I Can't Believe It's Not Butter® and other Trans Fat-Free spreads. These spreads should contain healthy monounsaturated fats and heart-healthy omega-3 fatty acids.

3. *Eat no fewer than 30 Grams of high fiber, complex good carbohydrate foods daily*, consisting of fruits, vegetables, nuts, beans, lentils, seeds, and whole-grain foods. Fruits and vegetables are allowed in almost unlimited quantities. These good carbohydrates have a low glycemic index that prevents spikes in insulin levels, which in turn causes sudden drops in blood sugar and results in fat being deposited in your fat cells. Concentrate on eating healthy whole grain breads, cereals, pasta, and other whole grains such as bran, wheat germ, bulgur, and whole grain rice, avocados, sweet potatoes, nuts, seeds, beans, and legumes. Consume at least 30 or more grams of fiber daily for good health and weight-loss.

- Sneak in the veggies and the fruits whenever possible. Most people don't get their three servings each of fruits and vegetables daily. The way to sneak in your daily allotment of fruits and vegetables is to add them to almost any food that you order or eat that doesn't come with fruits or vegetables included. For instance, get fruit (berries, bananas, peaches) on your low fat or whole wheat waffles or pancakes. Add green peppers, mushrooms, onions, broccoli, or spinach to your tomato pizza. Put salsa on your salad or sandwich. Use sliced apples, pears, and grapes in your salads. Put a sliced banana on your peanut butter sandwich. Order a veggie burger instead of a meat burger. Load up any sandwich with cucumbers, avocados, tomatoes, lettuce, and sprouts. In most cases within reason, you can *eat as many fresh fruits and vegetables (raw or steamed—no butter or oils added) as you'd like to eat.*

4. *Eliminate refined, so-called bad carbohydrates* from your diet, which include refined sugar, white flour, white rice and white pasta; processed and packaged foods; baked goods (pastries, biscuits, cookies, crackers, cakes, muffins, etc., that are made with trans-fats (hydrogenated or partially hydrogenated oils)). Refined sugar causes your blood sugar and insulin levels to peak, which in turn increases your appetite and stores unwanted fat deposits in your body.

5. The DietWalk Plan also adds *healthy lean protein* for increased energy, fitness and appetite control. Include beans, nuts, seeds, beans, lentils, and whole-grain products. Also, eat moderate amounts of other lean protein foods, consisting of low-fat dairy foods (milk, cheese, yogurt, tofu and soy), egg whites and other vegetable protein products. You can also to add low-fat lean non-vegetable protein to your diet, such as fish, and poultry without the skin, and occasionally very lean cuts of lamb, pork, veal and lean beef (small portions only with all of the fat trimmed off, once or twice a week).

- When you are on a low-calorie diet, your body needs more protein for the production of energy and your body's cell maintenance. Protein is the essential nutrient responsible for the maintenance and repair of all your organs, tissues, muscles, brain, and bones. All foods are sources of energy; however, protein provides a greater boost in energy levels since it is absorbed slowly and thus produces a constant source of energy.

- *Stay away from harmful protein.* Most high protein diets have you eating 3-4 times more protein than the recommended dietary allowance, and in most cases, the high protein you are eating is the harmful, high-fat protein. These diets tax your kidneys and leach out calcium from your bones, in addition to contributing to elevated blood cholesterol, heart disease, and strokes. Minimize fatty meats, fatty poultry with the skin intact and dairy products such as whole milk and butter, margarine, and vegetable oils (except olive, canola and peanut oils). Even though egg yolks are high in cholesterol, they are extremely low in saturated fat. Egg yolks have gotten a lot of bad press over the years because of their high cholesterol levels; however, 3 or 4 egg yolks per week can actually be beneficial because of their high content of protein, nutrients, and important antioxidants.

STEP 2: DIETWALK®: 30 MINUTE PLAN

The second step consists of 30 minutes of an aerobic exercise walking program six days per week for an additional calorie-burning power boost. Walking also produces a fresh supply of oxygen surging through your blood vessels to all of your body's tissues and cells. This walking plan boosts the weight-loss power of the DietWalk Plan by burning additional calories. This walking plan will also allow you to develop maximum cardiovascular physical fitness, good health and longevity.

Walking is the very best and safest aerobic exercise. Walking regularly helps your body deliver a steady supply of oxygen to all of your body's cells, tissues, and organs. This increased blood supply of oxygen to your body's cells keeps your body's metabolism in perfect balance and helps you to burn extra fat calories so that you can lose weight quickly and safely. Strenuous exercises can do considerably more harm than good.

When you exercise you burn more calories than you eat. It's not necessary to join a gym or participate in aerobics classes to burn up fat. You can burn calories by just climbing the stairs, cleaning the house, riding a bike, working in the garden, or just by walking 30 minutes every day. You don't even have to work up a sweat to burn calories while exercising. Studies have proven that people who take a brisk walk for 30 minutes every day burn body fat, improve their physical fitness, and lower their blood pressure, as much as, if not even more than, people who work out at a gym three to four days per week. Even two 15-minute walks per day will give you the same fitness and fat-burning benefits as one 30-minute walk every day.

A recent study from a major university showed that sedentary women, in addition to gaining weight in their abdomens, buttocks, and thighs, actually increased the amount of deep fat that surrounds the internal organs of the body. This increases the risk of heart disease, hypertension, and diabetes. The study also showed that moderate exercise five to six times per week for 30 minutes daily decreased the deep fat by more than 35% and resulted in considerable weight loss over a three-month period.

Step 3: Dietwalk: Body-Shaping Plan

The 3ʳᵈ step is the body-shaping plan, which includes the Diet-Walk Plan along with ***strength-training exercises.*** By adding weight-bearing exercises to your walking program you will in effect have a *double blast of metabolic calorie burning*, by combining an aerobic exercise with strength training exercises. Strength-training also builds muscles, strengthens bones, and boosts your metabolism. This is easily accomplished by using light-weight, hand-held weights during your 30-minute walk, three days per week. This plan, in addition to helping you lose weight, will actually sculpt and mold all of your body's muscles and give you a shapelier figure.

There is no need to do strenuous exercises or power weight lifting in order to get the perfect body. This diet and exercise walking program will help you to lose weight more quickly by burning additional calories. When you walk for 30 minutes using light-weight, hand-held weights, three days per week, you will develop maximum cardiovascular fitness, increased calorie burning for additional weight-loss, and body-shaping. This addition of weight-bearing exercises strengthens your bones, builds strong muscles, and boosts your metabolic rate. These strength-training exercises are what shape your body's muscles and figure. This double-blast of calorie burning from the aerobic effects of walking, combined with the additional calorie-burning from the strength-training exercise, is the final step that makes this weight loss plan so successful. The DIETWALK Plan will help you to slim down, shape up, and look younger, and you can actually lose up to 12 pounds in only 2 weeks.

CHAPTER ONE RAPID READ

STEP 1: DIETWALK® 30/30 PLAN.

- Eat no more than *30 grams of total fat* and no less than *30 grams of fiber* each day (see Fat & Fiber Counter in Chapter 10).

- Decrease unhealthy fats; increase healthy fats
  - Less fat taken in results in more storage fat being burned as fuel, resulting in more fat lost from your body, which results in steady, permanent weight loss.
  - The dietary fat calories can be stored in fat cells when you take in excess calories of fat in your diet–**it is the fat in your diet that makes you fat!**

- Eat high fiber, complex carbohydrates

- Eat lean proteins
  - Almost all the protein that you eat is burned as fuel for living

STEP 2: DIETWALK®: 30 MINUTE PLAN

- Slow, repetitious physical activity such as walking burns fat stored in the body, which is the best type of exercise for sustained weight loss.
- Spend 30 minutes six days per week walking for an additional calorie burning power boost.

STEP 3: DIETWALK: BODY-SHAPING PLAN

- Add strength-training exercises to your walking for a *double blast of metabolic calorie burning,*

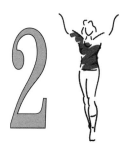

LOSE 12 POUNDS IN ONLY 2 WEEKS

The **DIETWALK Plan** consists of eating 30 grams of fat and 30 grams of fiber daily, combined with 30 minutes of walking six days per week. Weight loss is fast and easy, and what's more, it's permanent. There is no rebound weight gain, no food cravings, no starvation techniques, no liquid protein drinks, and no diet pills. There's no unhealthy low-carb diets to follow, where you end up stuffing your face with meat, eggs, cheese, butter, cream, bacon, fat and more fat, until you and your arteries are ready to explode. With the DietWalk plan you'll easily get rid of those unwanted pounds quickly and permanently.

The DietWalk Plan is specifically designed for women of all ages, all shapes, all sizes, and all weights. The weight loss plan is easy to follow and works quickly to shed all of the extra unwanted pounds that you want to lose. This easy plan is essentially a diet that is high in fiber, complex carbohydrates, and lean protein. This diet limits your intake of saturated fats, cholesterol, refined carbohydrates and sugars, and salt, caffeine, and alcohol. When combined with a 30-minute walk 6 days per week, you have a diet and exercise plan that has been proven to be permanently effective in weight loss, weight control, fitness, and good health.

QUICK WEIGHT LOSS FORMULA

1. Eat no more than 30 Grams of Total Fat Daily (concentrate on heart-healthy monounsaturated fats and reduce saturated fats)

2. Eat no less than 30 Grams of Fiber daily.

3. Do not eat refined or processed foods (sugar, white flour, and white rice). Do not eat packaged or commercially baked goods made with hydrogenated or partially hydrogenated oils.

4. Limit salt, caffeine and alcohol.

5. Drink at least six 8 oz. glasses of water daily.

6. Walk 30 minutes, six days per week.

DIETWALK: 30/30 MEAL PLANS

The basic diet is divided into easy to follow meal plans. Each of these daily diet meal plans have already been formulated to contain 30 grams of total fat and 30 grams fiber per day, without having to add up the number of grams of fat and fiber.

Once you've completed the first few weeks of your diet, these basic DietWalk Meal Plans will become an automatic part of your everyday schedule. The diet is extremely easy to follow. Once you've become comfortable with the basic meal plans, you can then start to formulate your own individual meals by eating no more than 30 grams of total fat and no less than 30 grams of fiber daily. You can mix and match any individual meal that you'd like.

There is such a variety of foods included in this 30/30 diet that your taste buds will never tire of this healthful, nutritious, palatable diet program. By varying the foods in your diet, there are never any hunger pangs or food cravings. Remember, that the DietWalk Plan in addition to controlling your weight, will add years to your life by providing essential, healthy nutrients, antioxidants, phyto-nutrients, vitamins and minerals, which eliminate harmful free-radical components from your body. This is a diet and exercise plan for fitness and health as well as for weight loss and body-shaping.

MONDAY

BREAKFAST

1 whole medium orange or ½ cup fresh orange juice

¾ cup cold whole grain or bran cereal with ½ cup any fresh fruit & ½ cup non-fat milk

1-2 cups coffee or tea (non-fat milk and artificial sweetener

LUNCH

1 cup soup (any type except cream based)—the more vegetables and beans, the better

whole wheat or multi-grain veggie sandwich with lettuce, tomatoes, sprouts, cucumber, carrots or any leafy green vegetable. Add Dijon mustard and sliced pickles.

1 glass decaffeinated sugar-free (coffee, tea, or soda)

8 oz. glass water

SNACK

1 medium orange or tangerine or handful of almonds or walnuts

8 oz. glass water

DINNER

Vegetable platter (broccoli, asparagus, squash, cauliflower, baked beans, carrots, green beans, spinach, mushrooms, stewed tomatoes, cauliflower)—choose any 4 (½ cup each)

1 whole-wheat dinner roll

4 oz. wine or 12 oz. light beer

8 oz. glass water

SNACK

½ cup raisins with 2 tbs. nuts (almonds, pecans or walnuts) -or- 1 cup mixed fresh fruit (strawberries, blueberries, blackberries purple grapes, etc.) -or- 1 high fiber, low fat oat and chocolate bar with ½ glass skim milk

8 oz. glass water

Total grams fat: 30.8 • Total grams fiber: 30.2
Walk 30 Minutes

TUESDAY

BREAKFAST

¾ cup cooked whole grain (oatmeal) *-or-* bran cereal with raisins (¼ cup) *-or-* any fresh fruit, cinnamon, ½ cup non-fat milk

1 medium orange *-or-* ½ cup orange juice

1-2 cups coffee or tea (non-fat milk, artificial sweetener)

LUNCH

1 slice pizza (tomato only or light cheese), topped with your choice of green peppers, mushrooms, onions, or garlic, etc..

1 large tossed salad with non-fat dressing

12 oz. diet drink of your choice (decaffeinated and sugar-free)

8 oz. glass water

SNACK

1 medium apple, pear, peach or nectarine and handful cashews

8 oz. glass water

DINNER

3 oz. baked eggplant or zucchini casserole parmesan baked with 1 tsp. olive oil and lightly breaded with whole wheat breading *-or-* 2 crumbled whole wheat crackers

1 cup steamed veggies (cauliflower, broccoli, spinach, etc.) and whole wheat roll

4 oz. tomato or vegetable juice and

8 oz. glass water

SNACK

½ cantaloupe or melon with ½ cup blueberries, strawberries or raspberries *-or-* 1 piece of fresh fruit (banana, pear, apple, peach, plum, orange or nectarine) s

8 oz. glass water

Total grams fat: 30.5 • Total grams fiber: 30.5

Walk 30 Minutes

WEDNESDAY

BREAKFAST	1 slice of whole wheat bread *-or-* whole wheat English muffin (½ teaspoon non-fat whipped/diet margarine without trans-fats or 1 tsp. jelly) 1 whole medium orange *-or-* 4 oz. (½ cup) fresh orange juice 1-2 cups coffee or tea (artificial sweetener & non-fat milk)
LUNCH	1 cup soup (vegetable, tomato, lentil, bean, pea, celery, minestrone, consommé, chicken noodle/rice, Manhattan clam chowder—no creamed or pureed soups). Low fat peanut butter and jelly sandwich on whole wheat muffin 1 cup decaffeinated sugar free (coffee, tea or diet soda) 8 oz. glass water
SNACK	Small box raisins and handful of walnuts 8 oz. glass water
DINNER	4 oz. tomato or V8 juice Tossed salad (lettuce, tomato, cucumber, carrots, celery) with lemon and/or 1 tsp olive oil and dash of vinegar dressing or 1 tsp. non-fat dressing 3 oz. whole-wheat pasta primavera (fresh veggies and ½ cup marinara sauce with or without mushrooms and garlic. Add small amount Parmesan cheese 1 whole wheat dinner roll 8 oz. glass water
SNACK	2 cups unbuttered, unsalted popcorn (hot air popcorn popper without oil) *-or-* 1 cup mixed fruits (berries, purple grapes, bananas) 8 oz. glass water

Total grams of fat: 30.1 • Total grams of fiber: 30.8

Walk 30 Minutes

THURSDAY

BREAKFAST

4 medium dried or stewed prunes -or- ½ cantaloupe or honey-dew melon -or- 1 cup any fresh fruit

1 slice whole or cracked wheat bread (½ teaspoon whipped/diet oil-free margarine or 1 tsp. jelly)

1-2 cups coffee or tea (artificial sweetener and non-fat milk)

LUNCH

1 cup fresh fruit salad on bed of lettuce with ½ cup low-fat cottage cheese and 2 whole-wheat crackers -or-

1 small chef salad with turkey (2 slices) and low-fat cheese (1 slice) only; use lemon, vinegar or 1 tsp. non-fat dressing

cup decaffeinated sugar free (coffee, tea or diet soda)

8 oz. glass water

SNACK

1 medium pear or handful walnuts or almonds

8 oz. glass water

DINNER

Large tossed salad (lettuce, tomato, celery, carrots, cucumber), with non-fat dressing

3 oz. broiled or baked chicken breast, skin removed; add seasoning (paprika, garlic, pepper, etc.)

½ cup brown long whole grain rice or ½ cup frozen corn or (1) small ear whole kernel corn (no butter, margarine, or salt)

1 cup steamed veggies (broccoli or spinach)

4 oz. tomato or vegetable juice

8 oz. glass water

SNACK

⅛ slice angel food cake with non-fat whipped cream and sliced fruit or berries -or- ½ cup low fat frozen yogurt or a high fiber, low fat cereal bar

8 oz. glass water

Total grams fat: 30.4 • Total grams fiber: 30.3

Walk 30 Minutes

FRIDAY

BREAKFAST

½ medium grapefruit 4 oz. (½ cup) fresh *-or-* unsweetened grapefruit juice

¾ cup cooked or cold whole grain (bran type) unsweetened cereal with ½ cup non-fat milk, ½ medium banana *-or-* 2 dozen raisins (½ oz.)

1-2 cups coffee or tea (artificial sweetener and non-fat milk)

8 oz. glass water

LUNCH

3 oz. (½ cup) tuna or chicken salad stuffed in whole-wheat pita bread (1 tsp. fat-free mayonnaise), with lettuce, tomato and cucumber. Use tuna packed in water.

1 cup decaffeinated sugar-free (coffee, tea or diet soda)

8 oz. glass water

SNACK

medium peach or banana and handful Brazil nuts

8 oz. glass water

DINNER

Large tossed salad with non-fat dressing (lettuce, tomato, celery, carrot, cucumber)

3 oz. baked or broiled fish (flounder, salmon, haddock, halibut, cod, sole, bass, bluefish, perch, trout) with lemon

1 medium baked potato or baked yam including skin (no butter, margarine or sour cream)

1 cup steamed vegetables (your choice)

4 oz. red wine or 12 oz. light beer

8 oz. glass water

SNACK

2 small unsalted, whole wheat pretzels or one medium soft pretzel (Superpretzel®) with or without mustard *-or-* ¾ cup non-fat yogurt or low-fat fruit cottage cheese with 2 tsp. wheat germ or Miller's bran

8 oz. glass water

Total grams of fat: 30.0 • Total grams of fiber: 29.6

Walk 30 Minutes

SATURDAY

BREAKFAST

2 eggs (egg white or artificial egg) omelet with tomato, green peppers, onions and any non-fat cheese *-or-* 1 poached or fried egg (non-fat, oil-free margarine—soft type)

½ cup orange or grapefruit juice

1 slice whole wheat, rye or pumpernickel bread with all fruit jam (1 T)

1- 2 cups coffee (non-fat milk, artificial sweetener)

LUNCH

1 cup soup any type except creamed—the more veggies and beans the better

Large tossed salad with ½ tsp. olive oil & vinegar or non-fat dressing

2 whole-wheat crackers

Diet drink of your choice (decaffeinated and sugar-free)

8 oz. glass water

SNACK

Any fruit or handful of walnuts or cashews *-or-* 1 baked apple (artificial sweetener) and cinnamon and raisins

8 oz. glass water

DINNER

3 oz. veal (lean) scaloppini or chicken (white meat without skin) cacciatore (baked with tomatoes, onions, peppers, mushrooms and garlic—your choice)

1 small baked or sweet potato with skin (no butter or sour cream)

1 slice whole wheat bread or roll

4 oz. tomato or vegetable juice

8 oz. glass water

SNACK

1 cup mixed fruit (berries, bananas, peach, grapes, kiwi, etc.) *-or-* ½ cup low fat frozen yogurt

8 oz. glass water

Total grams fat: 30.7 • Total grams fiber: 30.9

Walk 30 Minutes

SUNDAY

BREAKFAST

2 small whole grain pancakes (e.g., buckwheat made with egg substitute) topped with fresh fruit or sugar-free syrup

½ cup (4 oz.) orange juice or 1 medium orange

1-2 cups coffee or tea (non-fat milk, artificial sweetener)

LUNCH

Nicoise salad: tuna (dry), tomato, ½ sliced hard-boiled egg, (3) black olives, (1) anchovy, onion, bell pepper, radish and celery (balsamic vinaigrette dressing on the side—just a few fork-fulls)

Diet drink of your choice (decaffeinated and sugar-free)

8 oz. glass water

SNACK

1 small box raisins *-or-* ½ cup grapes (purple or green) with 6 almonds

8 oz. glass water

DINNER

3 oz. sirloin steak (lean) with grilled onions, mushrooms, garlic, peppers—your choice

1 medium baked potato *-or-* sweet potato with skin (no butter or sour cream)

1 cup steamed vegetables—your choice

4 oz. red wine or 12 oz. light beer

8 oz. glass water

SNACK

¾ cup sugar-free, fat-free ice cream *-or-* sugar-free Jell-O with non-fat whipped cream *-or-* High fiber, low fat, chocolate and oat bar

8 oz. glass water

Total grams fat: 28.8 • Total grams fiber: 30.1
REST!

After you have reached your ideal weight on this easy diet program, you will never again have to worry about rebound weight gain. The DietWalk: 30/30 plan enables you to lose weight quickly utilizing only these basic sample menu plans during your initial weight-loss program, or by following any of the optional meal plans, which are listed at the end the basic weekly meal plans.

OPTIONAL MEAL PLANS

The following lists are a variety of 30 Grams Fat / 30 Grams Fiber options for your meal plans. Each meal (breakfast, lunch & dinner) has already been pre-calculated to add up to approximately 1/3 of the allotted fat and fiber grams for each day. When you combine any three meals (breakfast, lunch & dinner), you'll have the total allotted 30 grams fat/30 grams fiber for any given day (for additional foods, see Fat & Fiber Counter in Chapter 10).

DIETWALK®: BREAKFAST OPTIONS

- 1 fried egg with non-fat spray and two small veggie non-fat sausages or two slices non-fat turkey bacon
- 1 fried egg with non-fat spray and 1 slice whole wheat bread and 1 tsp. all-fruit jam
- 1 non-fat waffle with fresh fruit topping
- Two small whole wheat or buckwheat pancakes made with egg substitute topped with fresh fruit and/or sugar free syrup
- 1 poached egg with 1 slice whole wheat toast and 1 tsp. all-fruit jam
- ½ cup low-fat granola with ½ cup blueberries and strawberries
- 1 scooped-out whole wheat bagel with 1 slice unsalted smoked salmon (nova lox), with non-fat cream cheese, tomato and onion
- 1 cup cold bran-type or whole wheat cereal with ½ cup any fresh fruit

- 2 egg whites or egg substitute omelet with 1 slice low-fat (skim milk) cheese, tomato, onions, green peppers, mushrooms (any or all)

- 1 cup cooked oatmeal or wheatena with cinnamon and ¼ cup raisins

- 1 cup fat-free yogurt with fresh fruit and 1T wheat germ

- 1 scrambled egg with non-fat spray and oat bran or whole wheat English muffin with 1 tsp. all-fruit jelly

- 1 toasted small whole wheat bagel with 1 tsp. non-fat cream cheese

- 1 slice cinnamon French toast with egg substitute and whole wheat bread

DIETWALK®: LUNCH OPTIONS

- 1 whole-wheat bun with two slices reduced-fat turkey breast, with lettuce, tomato, mustard or 1 tsp non-fat mayonnaise

- 1 cup Chinese greens with 6 medium grilled shrimp and garlic with 1 cup brown rice

- 1 non-fat cream cheese (2T) and jelly (2T) sandwich on whole wheat bread

- 1 whole-wheat bagel scooped out with 2 slices low-fat cheese, grilled with tomato and Dijon mustard or 1 tsp non-fat mayonnaise

- 1 whole wheat sandwich with two slices skim milk cheese (alpine lace) or other low-fat cheese, with lettuce, tomato, shredded carrots and sprouts, with mustard or 1 tsp. non-fat mayonnaise

- 1 small can fat-free baked beans, 1 non-fat beef hot dog or turkey dog on whole wheat bun with sauerkraut, relish and mustard and small side salad with 1 tsp non-fat dressing

- 2T non-fat cream cheese sandwich on whole wheat bread with sprouts, tomato, cucumber and lettuce 1 medium order steamed mussels or clams (12) with ½ cup marinara sauce with 1 small whole wheat roll

- 1 whole-wheat bagel scooped out with one slice smoked salmon (nova lox) with tomato, onion and lettuce

- 1 medium whole wheat pita pocket with grilled chicken breast (3 oz) and 1 tsp. non-fat mayonnaise with lettuce, tomato, celery and cucumber

- 1 T reduced-fat peanut butter & 1 T jelly sandwich whole wheat bread

- 1 soft corn tortilla with 1/3 cup fat-free refried beans with shredded low-fat cheese, lettuce, tomato and salsa

- ½ veggie hoagie (tomatoes, lettuce, olives, peppers, onions, cucumbers, carrots, sprouts-your choice) with roll scooped out leaving only shell of Italian roll

- 1 medium whole wheat pita pocket with tuna (3 oz) packed in water with lettuce, tomato, cucumber, sprouts and 1 tsp. Dijon mustard or 1 tsp. non-fat mayonnaise

- 1 veggie burger on whole wheat bread or bun with lettuce, tomato, onion & ketchup

- 1 cup soup (minestrone, lentil, split pea or any vegetable or bean-based soup) with one small whole-wheat roll

- 1 can (3 oz) sardines (drain oil) on whole wheat bread or pita with tomato, lettuce and onion

- Spinach salad with 1 oz low-fat blue cheese, ½ oz. chopped walnuts, sliced apples, cherry tomatoes, cucumbers, in 1 T dressing made with mustard, lemon and 1 tsp olive oil

- Panini sandwich toasted on scooped-out Italian or French roll with tomato, low-fat mozzarella cheese, basil and lettuce

- Nicoise salad with mixed greens, tuna, string beans, tomato, anchovies, ½ sliced hardboiled egg, olives, radishes, celery, onions and bell pepper with mustard vinaigrette dressing on on the side (dip fork in dressing sparingly) and one scooped out French roll

- Goat cheese salad with reduced-fat goat cheese, mixed greens, tomato, olives, bell peppers, cucumber, celery, with mustard vinaigrette dressing on the side (dip fork in dressing sparingly) and one scooped-out French roll

Dietwalk®: Dinner Options

- 2 soft tacos with non-fat refried beans, lettuce, tomato, onion, grated non-fat cheese with 3 oz. sliced grilled chicken and salsa

- 3 oz broiled or baked cod, halibut, mackerel or sole with grilled onions, peppers, mushrooms and tomatoes, with lemon, wine and seasonings, small whole wheat dinner roll and tossed salad (see above)

- 1 cup spinach fettuccini with fresh vegetables and ½ cup tomato or marinara sauce and large tossed salad (see above)

- Chicken Caesar salad with lettuce, tomato, chopped celery, cucumber and with 3 oz grilled chicken breast and non-fat parmesan cheese and 1T fat-free Caesar dressing

- 1 cup whole wheat spaghetti with 12 clams or mussels, garlic, 1/3 cup white wine, 1 tsp olive oil and seasoning and large tossed salad (see above)

- 1 grilled 3 oz lean hamburger on whole wheat roll with lettuce, tomato, onion and ketchup and 1 small white potato made into oven-baked French fries (slice into fries, spray nonstick pan with non-fat spray and bake on 400 degrees until crisp)

- 1 small can of sardines (drain oil) or tuna packed in water in large tossed salad of lettuce or romaine, tomato, cucumber, pepper, onion, sprouts, carrots and olives and 1 tsp non-fat dressing or mustard-vinaigrette dressing

- 1 slice pizza (tomato, or with light cheese and tomato) topped with veggies of your choice and a side salad with 1 tsp non-fat dressing

- 3 oz lean roast beef with horseradish and small baked potato or yam with skin, 1 cup steamed veggies and small whole wheat roll

- 1 cup low-fat macaroni and cheese with 1cup zucchini, diced tomatoes, onions and garlic and an ear of corn or a small sweet potato and steamed fresh carrots (½ cup)

- 6 medium cooked peeled shrimp with cocktail sauce and small ear of corn and 1 cup steamed asparagus, broccoli or spinach

- 3 oz. grilled salmon steak or salmon fillet with tomatoes, on-ions, peppers and garlic and small baked potato or yam and 1 cup steamed vegetable (your choice)

- 2 small lamb chops (trim fat) with 2 tsp. mint jelly and whole broiled tomato with 1 small baked sweet potato and tossed salad (see above)

CHAPTER TWO RAPID READ

- Eat no more than 30 Grams of Total Fat Daily (concentrate on heart-healthy monounsaturated fats and reduce saturated fats)

- Eat no less than 30 Grams of Fiber daily.

- Do not eat refined or processed foods (sugar, white flour, and white rice). Do not eat packaged or commercially baked goods made with hydrogenated or partially hydrogenated oils.

- Limit salt, caffeine and alcohol.

- Drink at least six 8 oz. glasses of water daily.

- Always check the labels when buying food.

- Watch portion sizes and food preparation methods, especially when eating out.

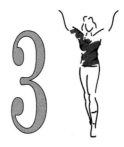

FEARLESS FIBER: SECRET AGENT

The DIETWALK Plan has a secret agent called **Fearless Fiber**, who is actually working for your health. This fiber secret agent blocks fat and burns calories for weight-loss, and also contains a multitude of healthy ingredients that prevent many degenerative diseases, including heart disease, high blood pressure, strokes, and some forms of cancer. This fiber agent actually helps us to live longer, healthier lives. Fearless Fiber is truly a hero and will help your body shed those unwanted pounds quickly and easily.

Fiber is the general term for those parts of plant food that we are unable to digest. Approximately 15% of the starch in foods (known as resistant starch) is tightly bound to fiber and resists the normal digestive processes. Bacteria normally present in the colon ferment this resistant starch and change it into short-chain fatty acids, which are important to normal bowel health and may also help to protect the colon from cancer-causing agents. Foods that contain resistant starch include breads, cereals, pasta, rice, potatoes, and legumes. Fiber is not found in foods of animal origin (meats and dairy products). Plant foods contain a mixture of different types of fibers. These fibers can be divided into soluble or insoluble depending on their solubility in water.

1. **Insoluble fibers:** (cellulose, hemi-celluloses, lignin) make up the structural parts of the cell walls of plants. These fibers absorb many times their own weight in water, creating a soft bulk to the stool and hasten the passage of waste products out of the body. These insoluble fibers promote bowel regularity and aid in the prevention and treatment of some forms of constipation, hemorrhoids, and diverticulitis. These insoluble fibers also may decrease the risk of colon cancer by diluting potentially harmful substances, particularly bile acids, which can cause inflammation and pre-cancerous changes in the lining of the wall of the colon. Insoluble fibers are found in barley, wheat bran, and other whole grains.

2. **Soluble fibers**: (gums, pectins, and mucilages) are found within the plant cells. These fibers form a gel, which slows both stomach emptying and absorption of simple sugars from the intestines. This process helps to regulate blood sugar levels, which is particularly helpful in diabetic patients and is helpful in controlling weight in non-diabetics. Many soluble fibers can also assist in lowering blood cholesterol by binding with bile acids and cholesterol and eliminating the cholesterol through the intestinal tract before the cholesterol can be absorbed into the bloodstream. These soluble fibers actually form a fiber network, like a spider's web, around fatty foods and carry them out of the intestines before they have a chance to be absorbed. Less fat absorbed means lower blood cholesterol and less fat deposited in your body's fat cells. The best sources of soluble fiber are fruits and vegetables, oat bran, barley, dried peas and beans, flax and psyllium seeds.

TWO SECRET AGENTS FIGHT FAT

Both soluble and insoluble fibers are important in a healthy diet. Your diet should contain at least 30 grams of fiber daily and at least ½ soluble fiber and ½ insoluble fiber. Both types of fiber help to lower fats in the bloodstream, particularly the bad form of cholesterol known as LDL cholesterol. Insoluble fiber helps to transport cholesterol out of the intestinal tract before it can be absorbed into the bloodstream. Soluble fiber helps to break down fats like cholesterol in the intestine so that when they are absorbed they are harmless fats.

New studies have shown that eating more *soluble fiber* found in oranges, apples, figs, and avocados can boost your immune system's cells to fight off bacterial and viral infections. Soluble fiber appears to increase the anti-inflammatory properties of your body's immune cells. Recent research has shown that soluble fiber boosts the body's production of a protein called *interleukin-4*, which stimulates your body's infection-fighting T-cells.

HOW FIBER HELPS YOU LOSE WEIGHT

Weight control is aided by the slower emptying of the stomach when you ingest soluble fibers. This causes a feeling of fullness and a decrease in hunger, causing fewer calories to be consumed. For example, if you eat an apple, which has a high fiber content, you'll have a feeling of fullness, as compared to eating a cupcake, which has no fiber, and which is the same weight and size as the apple. In fact, it would take approximately three cupcakes to satisfy your brain's hunger center before you realized that you were full. Well, by then you would already have consumed 480 calories and 17 grams of fat.

A. Fiber helps in weight loss and weight control by the simple fact that high-fiber foods contain **fewer calories for their large volume.** Fiber-rich foods, such as fruits and vegetables, whole grain cereals and breads, potatoes and legumes are low in fat calories and have high water content. You are, therefore, eating less and enjoying it more.

B. High fiber foods have a **high bulk ratio**, which satisfies the hunger center more quickly than low fiber foods; consequently, fewer calories are consumed. Fiber-rich foods take longer to chew and to digest than fiber-depleted foods, which, in turn gives your stomach time to feel full. Feeling full earlier leads to consuming fewer calories.

C. Foods with **high fiber content** are considerably **less concentrated in calories**. The following carbohydrate foods have a *low glycemic index*, and for all intents and purposes can be labeled as good carbs:

- Most vegetables, with the exception of corn and white potatoes.

- Most fruits with the skin intact, with the exception of fruit juices, which contain high levels of sugar and very little actual fruit. Some fruits, for example, watermelon and grapes, do have a high sugar content and have to be consumed in moderation.

- Beans and legumes are excellent sources of fiber, protein, vitamins, minerals, and nutrients.

- Whole grains:

  - Whole-grain cereals, such as oatmeal (instant oatmeals may have a high sugar content) or cold cereals are good choices for low glycemic carbohydrates. Make sure that the package shows a fiber count of at least 5 to 6 grams of fiber or more per serving, and a sugar count lower than 10 to 12 grams of sugar per serving, preferably less than 8 grams.

  - Whole-grain breads. The label on whole-grain breads should show that the first ingredient listed is "whole grain flour." If it doesn't list whole-grain flour first, then it is really not a whole-grain bread. This includes any type of whole-grain bread products.

  - Brown long-grain rice makes a good low glycemic addition to any meal, since it is broken down and absorbed slowly.

  - Whole wheat pastas now come in many varieties, such as noodles, spaghetti, vermicelli, linguini, etc.

- Nuts are good low glycemic snack foods. In addition to being absorbed slowly, they are excellent sources of protein, fiber, magnesium, copper, folic acid, potassium, and vitamin D. Nuts are also considered to be "the good fats," which are actually called monosaturated fats. They help to keep the blood vessels open, which, in turn, can reduce the risk of heart disease and strokes. Raw nuts, in particular, are called "heart healthy" nuts, since they contain generous amounts of omega-3 fatty acids. These omega-3 fatty acids are heart protective, and have also been known to prevent certain forms of cancer.

D. A high-fiber diet is essentially a **healthy, low-fat diet**, which decreases the intake of refined and processed food. This encourages the consumption of fresh fruits, vegetables, and whole-grain cereals and breads. When fiber is eaten from food sources, it produces its most beneficial effect, especially when it is eaten with each meal of the day. Dietary fiber takes longer to chew and eat, with the subsequent development of more saliva and a larger bulk swallow with each mouthful. High-fiber diets help to provide bulk without energy and may reduce the amount of energy absorbed from the food that is eaten. These high-fiber diets are often referred to as having a low-energy density and appear to prevent excessive caloric (energy) intake. Countries that consume high-fiber diets rarely have obesity problems. The DietWalk Plan incorporates at least 30 grams or more of fiber into its diet for good health and weight-loss.

E. High fiber good carbs **burn more calories during digestion** and make you feel fuller earlier **and longer** than eating refined bad carbs. These good carbs have **a low glycemic index** and are absorbed slowly and cause only a moderate rise in blood sugar and insulin levels. This even level of insulin can **slowly process the blood sugar into the body's cells for energy production** and there is no rapid filling of the cells with fat caused by high levels of sugar and insulin surges, which in turn, causes binge carbohydrate eating. Most vegetables (except corn and white potatoes), fruits (not fruit juices), beans, nuts, legumes, chick peas, brown rice, popcorn, whole-grain cereals and breads fall into this category. The good carbs are primarily of plant origin and are naturally low in fat and calories, and contain phyto-nutrients, vitamins, minerals, enzymes and fiber. Many of these good carbohydrates actually contain protein as well.

These good carbs are helpful in a weight-loss program because your body slowly converts these good carbs into glucose in the intestinal tract, which is then slowly absorbed into the bloodstream. This results in your appetite being nicely controlled and prevents you from gaining excess weight gain.

F. Both fiber and protein help to curb your appetite by helping you to feel fuller earlier in the course of your meal. This fiber-protein combo slows the rate at which your body absorbs this combination of protein and fiber, thus minimizing blood sugar and insulin spikes, which can otherwise stimulate your appetite. Also by preventing the production of excess insulin, this fiber-protein combo prevents fat from being deposited in your fat cells, particularly those fat cells located in your abdominal wall. So, in effect, you are melting away belly fat as you consume this important fiber-protein combination.

By increasing the lean protein content and decreasing the fat content of your meals, you can slowly and safely lose weight that will stay permanently lost. Unlike low-carb, high-fat diets, you won't experience rapid rebound weight gain that invariably occurs when you stop the diet, and you'll avoid the nasty side effects and hidden health problems inherent in these unsafe low-carb diets. All low carb diets are high-fat diets and the excess fat calories you eat are stored in your fat cells indefinitely. Complex carbs, on the other hand, cause your body to work harder during digestion, burning more calories for immediate energy production and for glycogen storage in your muscles and liver for later use.

FIBER BLOCKS FATS AND BURNS CALORIES

Dietary fiber is one of your best foods to block both the absorption of fat and to burn up extra calories. Sounds almost too good to be true; however, it really works. First of all, when you combine the high-fiber foods that we have already discussed, combined with any fat in your diet, like a piece of cake or a hamburger, each gram of fiber traps fat globules by entwining them in a fiber-like web, made up of thousands of fiber strands. Once these fat globules are trapped in the fiber's web, they pass through the intestinal tract before they are absorbed into the bloodstream. Therefore, these fat globules are excreted in the waste material from your colon without getting absorbed and stored as fat in your body. The fiber is actually removing the fat from your body like a garbage truck removes garbage. And to underscore that fact, fat really is garbage.

Secondly, fiber actually burns up calories by itself. This is accomplished because fiber causes your intestinal tract to work harder in order to digest the fiber foods. The body's metabolism therefore uses more energy for this time-consuming digestion, and therefore can actually consume most of the calories that the fiber foods contain. Strange as it seems, some heavily fibered foods can actually burn up more calories than the fiber foods contain, thereby creating a deficit of calories. This causes the body to use stored body fat for the production of energy. Each gram of fiber that you consume can burn up approximately 9 calories, most of which come from fat. So, if you eat 30 grams of fiber a day, you can actually burn up an additional 270 calories daily (30 grams fiber x 9 calories). You can actually subtract those 270 calories every day from your total daily calorie intake, without actually cutting those calories from your diet. In addition to blocking fat and burning calories, fiber foods bind with water in the intestinal tract and form bulk that makes you feel full early in the course of your meal. So, you eat less, and therefore you consume fewer calories at each meal. Also, your appestat (hunger mechanism) is satisfied for longer periods of time, since it takes longer to digest fiber foods, and therefore you will have less of a tendency to snack between meals.

HEALTHY COLORS OF THE FOOD SPECTRUM

Many recent medical studies have proved that colorful fruits and vegetables and grains, nuts and seeds, contain cancer-fighting substances and can provide a full spectrum of disease prevention. For maximum health benefits, you should eat a variety of vegetables and fruits of many different colors. These colors are formed by pigments in each individual plant. The reason for the different colors is that each colored fruit or vegetable has a different phyto-chemical (phyto means plant). These phyto-chemicals in the fruits and vegetables contain many essential nutrients that help to decrease the risk of heart disease, hypertension, blood clots, degenerative diseases of aging, and certain forms of cancer. It is important to eat at least 4-5 servings of fruit or vegetables per day. The DietWalk Plan contains an abundance of all of these healthy nutrients.

The following is a list of some of the phyto-chemicals and antioxidants present in fruits, vegetables, grains and seeds and nuts that can reduce your risk of many diseases such as cancer and heart disease:

VEGETABLES

Spinach If you're looking for a vegetable with super healing powers, try spinach. It's packed with vitamins, antioxidants, and minerals that will protect you from many diseases. Spinach contains many antioxidants including beta and alpha carotenes, lutein, zeaxanthin, potassium, magnesium, vitamin K and folic acid. Recent studies at two major universities have found that, as strange as it seems, spinach may lower the risk of strokes, colon cancer, cataracts, heart disease, osteoporosis, hip fractures, memory loss, Alzheimer's disease, depression and even birth defects. The disease fighting properties in spinach are better absorbed when spinach is cooked with a little olive oil. Now, that's what I call a power vegetable.

Other dark green leafy vegetables (collard greens, kale, bok choy, mustard greens) are low in calories and have high fiber content. These crunchy foods take longer to chew, which helps to shut off the brain's hunger control mechanism (appestat). This fiber also prevents the absorption of fat from the gastro-intestinal tract by wrapping thread like fibers around the fat globules, and quickly eliminates them out of the intestinal tract, before they have a chance to be absorbed.

Kale and spinach are two vegetables rich in the antioxidants *lutein* and *zeaxanthin*. These antioxidants have been reported to protect against age-related cataracts and macular degeneration, one of the leading causes of blindness. Also, high in these vision-protecting antioxidants are romaine lettuce, broccoli, collards, turnip greens, and corn.

Green leafy vegetables are low in calories and are filling because of their fiber content and their crunch factor. Crunchy fiber foods take longer to eat and help your brain's hunger mechanism to shut down quickly. Green leafy vegetables also contain many plant nutrients, antioxidants, and B-complex vitamins, which help to prevent cancer, heart disease, and degenerative neurological diseases.

Broccoli and Brussels sprouts also contain power nutrients that can reduce your risk of heart disease, and certain types of cancer. The active antioxidant in broccoli is *glucoraphanin*, which has been shown to boost your body's defense mechanism against cancer-causing free radicals which damage normal cells in the body. This particular antioxidant also lowers blood pressure, strengthens the immune system, decreases inflammation in the body and has been shown to reduce the incidence of strokes.

Cruciferous vegetables also decrease risk of bladder cancer. In a recent study on bladder cancer, it was shown that in order to reduce the risk of bladder cancer, it is necessary to drink lots of fluids, not to smoke, and to eat lots of cruciferous vegetables. A high intake of cruciferous vegetables, particularly broccoli and cabbage, significantly reduced the risk of bladder cancer. This may be explained by the presence of one or more phytochemicals in broccoli and cabbage, which are specific in the reduction of bladder cancer risk. This study also showed that a high intake of fruits, yellow vegetables, and green, leafy vegetables did not significantly reduce the risk of bladder cancer. The relationship with high cruciferous vegetable intake (broccoli and cabbage) was associated with the highest reduction in the risk of developing bladder cancer.

Sweet Potatoes are excellent sources of folic acid, beta-carotene, potassium, vitamins A C, B-complex and beta-carotene. These nutrients combined with sweet potatoes plant sterols can decrease your risk of heart disease. When eaten with the skin they are an excellent source of both soluble and insoluble fiber and are great for your Diet-Step: 30/30 weight-loss plan.

Contrary to popular belief, sweet potatoes are excellent sources of vitamins and minerals and are considered good carbs. They are a great addition to any weight-loss program because of their high fiber content and their nutritional value. Sweet potatoes are good sources of vitamin C, B-complex, folic acid, potassium, vitamin A, and beta-carotene. These nutrients combined with plant sterols, found in sweet potatoes, are powerful antioxidants, which can help to lower cholesterol and lower your risk of heart disease. When sweet potatoes are eaten with their skin, they are good sources of both insoluble and soluble fiber. These two types of fibers help to reduce your appetite the way most fiber foods do, by filling you up and satisfying your appetite early, without supplying extra calories in your diet.

Tomatoes contain the antioxidant lycopene which helps to prevent both prostate and breast cancers. Tomatoes also contain lots of vitamin C, which when combined with *lycopene* can help to lower your blood cholesterol. Tomatoes also contain an amino acid called caritine, which helps you to lose weight, by increasing your metabolic rate, which in turn burns fat calories faster.

Tomatoes are unique in their ability to produce an amino acid called *carnitine*. This amino acid causes your body to burn fat at a faster rate by increasing your body's basal metabolic rate. Any tomato products, from ketchup to tomato sauce, are great for your weight-reducing diet. Tomatoes also contain abundant amounts of vitamin C and an antioxidant called lycopene, which helps to prevent several types of cancer, including breast and prostate cancers. The combination of vitamin C and lycopene also helps to prevent the buildup cholesterol in your bloodstream.

Asparagus contains a unique antioxidant called glutathione, which helps to fight dangerous free-radicals, which in turn can damage normal cells in your body. Asparagus is a good source of folic acid, potassium, beta-carotene, vitamin C and fiber. Asparagus is an excellent source of potassium, folic acid, beta-carotene, vitamin C, and the antioxidant *glutathione*, which helps to fight nasty free radicals, which can damage normal cells. Asparagus is a great addition to any diet program, since it is low in calories and high in nutrients. Steamed asparagus is great eaten alone or in a salad. It must be refrigerated or frozen quickly to prevent the loss of its nutritional value. If boiled too long, most of the nutrients end up in the water.

Beans are high in potassium and low in sodium, which helps to reduce your risk of developing high blood pressure and strokes Beans are chock full of fiber, which helps to reduce the absorption of fat and unwanted calories from the gastro-intestinal tract. The high fiber content of beans is great for your weight loss plan, since it reduces your appetite by filling you up faster, so that you eat fewer calories. Beans have almost as many calories and as much protein as meat without the added saturated fat. The fiber and water content of beans make you feel fuller earlier in your meal so that you don't consume excess calories. One cup of cooked beans (⅔ of a can) contains 12 grams of fiber, whereas meat contains no fiber at all. Meat is therefore digested quickly whereas fiber is digested slowly, keeping you satisfied longer. Beans are also low in sugar, which prevents insulin from spiking in the bloodstream and causing hunger pangs.

The high fiber content of beans helps to reduce the absorption of both fat and calories from the intestinal tract. The fiber content of beans reduces your appetite and lets you eat fewer calories because you get filled up earlier. Beans are also high in potassium and low in sodium, which helps to reduce the risk of high blood pressure and strokes. Beans, beans—they're good for the heart, the more you eat them, the more you're smart!

In a recent study, bean eaters weighed on average, seven pounds less and had slimmer waists than their bean-avoiding counterparts. Beans also contain antioxidants and phytonutrients which fight dangerous free-radicals in your body, which can cause degenerative diseases of aging, cardiovascular diseases, and cancer. The beans that contained the most antioxidants were red kidney beans, pinto beans, small red beans, navy beans, black beans, and black-eyed peas. Beans have lots of fiber and protein and no fat at all. The perfect combo for a super power food.

Peas are packed with vitamins A, B-1, B-6, C, and vitamin K which is known for maintaining strong bones and helping blood to clot in order to prevent bleeding. Peas are high in fiber and are an excellent source of vegetable protein. They also have the added benefit of containing no fat or cholesterol. One cup of peas which contains approximately 100 calories has as much protein as a tablespoon of peanut butter or a 1/4 of a cup of nuts. Peas are another example of a super power food even though they're very small. Size doesn't really matter. Other vegetables that are rich sources of Vitamin K are cabbage, broccoli, spinach, cauliflower, and beans.

Peppers are great sources of vitamins A, C, B-complex, beta-carotene, folic acid and potassium. All colors of sweet peppers (red, yellow, green) are high in fiber and low in calories and are great foods for your Diet Walk weight-loss plan. Peppers contain spices that also can reduce your appetite because they satisfy your taste buds and hunger before you've had a chance to eat a big meal.

Peppers also have antioxidants that help to prevent strokes and heart attacks by decreasing the blood platelets' stickiness, thus preventing blood clots from forming. Hot peppers also contain antioxidants that help to prevent some forms of cancer. These hot peppers also contain a compound called *capsaicin*, which in addition to making the peppers taste hot, has anti-inflammatory properties, which helps to relieve the pain of arthritis and nerve inflammation. Red and green and yellow sweet peppers are excellent sources of vitamin C, vitamin A, and beta-carotene, B-complex vitamins, potassium, and folic acid. Since they are low in calories and high in fiber, peppers are excellent foods to add to your weight-loss program. Peppers contain antioxidants that help to prevent blood clots by decreasing the blood platelet's stickiness. This property can help to prevent heart attacks and strokes.

Hot peppers contain higher quantities of antioxidants than sweet peppers. They also contain phytonutrients that help to prevent certain forms of cancer. Hot peppers also contain an ingredient called capsaicin, which makes these peppers hot and spicy. This ingredient has anti-inflammatory properties and helps to relieve the pain of various forms of arthritis and nerve inflammation. These capsaicinoids can cause eye irritation if transferred from your hands to your eyes, so be careful to wash your hands thoroughly after handling hot peppers.

Soybeans contain soy proteins, which helps to reduce the risk of cardiovascular disease. The reason for this is that soy proteins reduce the amount of total fat and LDL cholesterol in the blood by affecting the synthesis and metabolism of cholesterol in the liver. Its amino acid composition differs from the structure of other proteins found in meat and milk. Clinical trials showed a significantly lower incidence of coronary heart disease in patients with a high soy intake. Soybeans can be found in many different varieties, including soy beverages, tofu, tempeh, soy-based meat substitutes, and some baked goods. However, to qualify, such soy-rich foods should contain at least 6.5 grams of soy protein, and less than 3 grams of total fat per serving and less than 1 gram of saturated fat per serving in order to qualify as a heart healthy food. One-half cup of cooked soybeans contains 4 grams of fiber. Soybeans are also a good source of dietary fiber.

In another related study, soy supplements were shown to cut the risk of developing colon cancer in half. Soy supplements also decreased the relative risk of having a recurrence of colon cancer in high-risk subjects. This study was reported at the annual conference of The American Institute for Cancer Research. High soy intake may be able to delay the onset of colon cancer in those at risk, or may lead to more cancer-free years in those whose initial cancer was surgically removed.

Soy contains natural phytonutrients called *isoflavones*. These plant chemicals break down the fat which is stored in your body's fat cells. Several studies have confirmed that the consumption of soy products on a regular basis helps dieters burn fat and lose weight without any other alteration in their diets. These isoflavones present in soy also have been shown to reduce the incidence of heart disease. In addition to helping you lose weight by breaking down the stored fat in your body, isoflavones also break down saturated fat in your blood, thus lowering the LDL bad cholesterol. Soy products (soy milk, soy yogurt, tofu, etc.) are good for heart and great for your figure.

Mushrooms: Many types of mushrooms contain the amino acid glutamic acid, which boosts the immune system and helps to fight various types of infections. By helping to improve the body's immune system, mushrooms have also been known to fight certain forms of cancer and autoimmune diseases, such as rheumatoid arthritis, lupus, and other collagen disease. Mushrooms are also rich in potassium and vitamin C, which help to keep blood pressure normal.

Portobello and white mushrooms have a high content of certain nutrients and minerals, particularly *selenium*, which may help to reduce the risk of prostate and breast cancer. When selenium is combined with the vitamin E present in mushrooms, it helps to prevent nasty free radicals from damaging the body's normal cells, thus slowing the aging process. Shiitake mushrooms also contain many plant nutrients, in particular *lentinan* and *eritadenine*, which help to improve the immune system and assist in lowering blood cholesterol. These phytonutrients have also been shown to reduce the risk of heart disease and certain forms of cancer.

All mushrooms are low in calories and are fat-free, making them excellent staples in a weight-loss program. They are excellent flavor enhancers for a variety of foods. Mushrooms are not only good for you, but they are great for your weight-loss program.

Onions and Curry: In a recent study from Johns Hopkins University School of Medicine, it was found that the chemicals found in onions and curry may help to prevent colon cancer. The antioxidant found in onions is called *quercetin*, and the antioxidant found in curry is called curcumin. It is thought that these two powerful antioxidants decrease the formation of colon polyps in patients who have an inherited-type of precancerous colon polyps. The average number of polyps decreased by 60% and the average size of the polyps decreased by 50% in patients who consumed these two powerful antioxidants found in both onions and curry.

FRUITS

Grapefruit contains high levels of potassium, vitamin C, beta-carotene, and the antioxidant *lycopene*, which has been shown to reduce the risk of both breast and prostate cancers. Grapefruits also contain bioflavonoids, which appear to protect against heart disease. They also contain phytonutrients, which include phenolic acid, which can block nitrosamines, which are cancer-causing chemicals found in many smoked foods.

Grapefruits are a great addition to any weight-reduction program, since they are low in calories and high in fiber. The only precaution is that patients who are on cholesterol-lowering drugs called the statins should be careful about drinking grapefruit juice with these medications. Grapefruit juice appears to slow the natural breakdown of these drugs in the bloodstream, causing higher than expected levels of these medications to stay active in the blood for longer periods of time. It is important for any patient on statin medication to check with their doctor before combining grapefruit with these cholesterol-lowering drugs.

Oranges protect your heart and fight cancer. In a recent study, it was shown that oranges boost HDL cholesterol, in addition to providing vitamin C, folic acid, and numerous flavonoids. These compounds are thought to prevent cholesterol oxidation, which has been linked to a reduced risk of coronary events. An orange or two a day will keep atherosclerosis away. Researchers have found that citrus fruits, in particular oranges, also showed anti-cancer activity in animals and in test tubes. These researchers found that animals that ate oranges for several months were 25% less likely to develop early colon cancer than animals given only water. Compounds such as *liminoids* in oranges seem to alter the characteristics of the colon lining, discouraging cancer growth. These researchers speculate that the orange juice may also help to suppress breast cancer, prostate, and lung cancer.

Blueberries may reverse the aging process. New research has indicated that women on antioxidant-rich diets showed fewer age-related disorders than those on a normal diet. The studies showed that among

all the fruits and vegetables, the benefits were greatest with blueberries, which reversed age-related effects; for example, loss of balance
and lack of coordination. They also discovered that blueberry extract
had the greatest effect on reversing aging decline. Antioxidants help
neutralize free radical by-products on the conversion of oxygen into
energy, which, if not neutralized, can cause oxidative stress and lead
to cell damage. Previous studies have shown that both strawberries
and spinach extract can also help to prevent the onset of age-related
defects. However, the greatest effect was shown in patients who ate
blueberries. Phytonutrients in blueberries, particularly flavonoids and
beta-carotene, seem to have an anti-inflammatory effect, which may
even help in the prevention of Alzheimer's disease. Again, we have
another solid recommendation for eating fruits and vegetables because of their high fiber content and because of their phytonutrients
and antioxidants.

Apples: The old adage that "an apple a day keeps the doctor
away" may contain more truth than we actually realize. When you eat
an apple with the skin on it every day, you help prevent many health-
related problems. Apples contain a mysterious antioxidant called
Quercetin which has many beneficial properties. First of all, this compound acts as an antihistamine which may help to relieve the symptoms of asthma and other allergy related problems. Quercetin also has
anti-inflammatory properties that may reduce the pain associated with
arthritis and other inflammatory problems. This unique antioxidant
has also been shown to protect the brain cells from circulatory damage, which can help to prevent strokes and reduce the incidence of
age-related neurological disorders such as Alzheimer's disease. And
finally, Quercetin has been shown to prevent certain forms of cancer,
including breast and prostate cancer.

Fruits and vegetables in general contain various healthy antioxidants and phytonutrients that prevent many cardiovascular and degenerative diseases of aging, including several forms of cancer. New
studies have also shown that fruits can prevent or reduce the incidence of uterine fibroids, which are the most commonly diagnosed

uterine tumors. These tumors have been associated with anemia, pelvic pain, and in some cases, fertility problems. It appears that women who have high levels of estrogens, which may be related to high meat intake, are more prone to fibroids. A recent study showed that diets decreasing or eliminating meats and increasing green vegetables have a significant effect on the prevention of the development of fibroids. The vegetables and fruits contain isoflavinoids, which can offset the effect of estrogen on the body. Also, by eliminating meat from the diet, the levels of estrogen in the body decrease. By decreasing meat and increasing fiber, the body is less likely to develop estrogen-related uterine fibroid tumors.

Veggies and fruits also help prevent breast and uterine cancer. Women who limit their intake of red meat and eat lots of green vegetables have a reduced risk of developing breast cancer and uterine cancer. High levels of estrogen, which results from the consumption of beef, ham, pork, and other red meat, have been implicated in the formation of breast and uterine cancer. The intake of 4-5 servings of fruits and vegetables daily with phytonutrients, in particular, isoflavinoids, may offset some of estrogen's effect on the uterus and breast.

In a recent study reported in the *Journal of the American Medical Association*, it appears that people who eat foods that are high in *plant-based estrogen* appear to have a lower incidence of lung cancer. Broccoli, cabbage, soy products, spinach and chick peas are excellent sources of plant based estrogens. Vegetables in general are low in calories and high in fiber, making them excellent choices for a healthy weight-loss program.

NUTS, SEEDS, AND GRAINS

Nuts have a low glycolic index and are absorbed slowly. They are also a good source of protein and contain many essential nutrients such as fiber, copper, magnesium, folic acid, vitamin D and E, and potassium. Nuts, particularly walnuts and almonds, contain heart-healthy monounsaturated fats. These good fats can lower blood cholesterol, prevent heart disease and reduce the incidence of high blood pressure. Nuts actually help to retain the natural elasticity of blood vessels which helps to lower blood pressure. Nuts, especially walnuts have a high content of an amino acid called L-argentine and also contain alpha-lanoline acid, which is a plant-based omega-3 fatty acid. These two compounds help to dilate your arteries and offer additional heart-protective properties as well as to help prevent certain forms of cancer.

Nuts are also an excellent source of protein, which act as a natural appetite suppressant because of its slow digestion and absorption into the bloodstream. Most of the energy contained in the protein in nuts is burned as fuel for all of your body's metabolic functions. Therefore, hardly any of the calories contained in the dietary protein found in nuts is converted into fat storage, which is why nuts are a good addition to the DietWalk weight-loss plan.

Frequent consumption of walnuts (four to five servings per week) has been shown to reduce the risk of coronary heart disease by as much as 50%. Nuts also have been shown to decrease both total cholesterol by 5-10% and LDL cholesterol by 15-20%. A study published in *The Journal of Nutrition* indicated that of all edible plants, walnuts have one of the highest concentrations of antioxidants. In a more recent study reported in the *Journal of Circulation*, from the Hospital Clinic of Barcelona, Spain, it was reported that this was the first time a whole food, not its isolated components, was shown to have beneficial effect on vascular health, and also that walnuts differ from all other nuts because of their high content of alpha-linolenic acid (ALA), a plant-based omega-3 fatty acid, which may provide additional heart-protective properties. Several other beneficial components of walnuts include *L-arginine*, which may be cardio protective by dilating the arteries. Walnuts also contain fiber, folic acid, gamma-tocopherol, and other antioxidants, which also help to prevent atherosclerosis (hardening of the arteries).

Nuts are packed with nutrition. They contain vitamin E, B-complex, folic acid, fiber, omega-3 fatty acids, and arginine (an amino acid). These nutrients contained in nuts have been shown to reduce blood cholesterol, prevent heart disease and stroke and protect the heart against irregular heart rhythms and help to maintain your blood vessels natural elasticity

Walnuts differ from other nuts because of their high content of *alpha-linolenic acid* (ALA), a plant-based omega-3 fatty acid, which may provide additional heart-protective properties.

Sunflower Power: Sunflower seeds contain many healthy nutrients including healthy monounsaturated fatty acids. These seeds are excellent sources of B vitamins: thiamine, folate, and pantothenic acids, and the minerals copper, zinc, iron, and selenium.

One ounce of sunflower seeds daily can improve your diet by providing all of these essential vitamins and minerals in addition to the heart-protective antioxidant vitamin E. Sunflower seeds and oil contain both mono and polyunsaturated fats which can reduce LDL (bad cholesterol) and increase beneficial HDL (good cholesterol) in the blood.

Whole grains: In a recent study in the *American Journal of Clinical Nutrition*, women who ate three to four servings of whole grains a day had one-third to one-half the risk of developing heart disease as opposed to women who ate refined flour, such as white bread. It is important to check the ingredients in any commercial food to see that it is truly made from whole grains. In particular, it is important to check the ingredients in snack foods (for example, cookies, crackers, and chips), since many of these products contain not only refined white flour, but also partially hydrogenated oils (trans-fats), which actually can raise our cholesterol more than other types of saturated fats.

Recent studies have subsequently shown that high fiber diets, which include not only cereal grains, but fruits and vegetables, do, indeed, help to prevent against the development of colon cancer. As part of the ongoing Nurses' Health Study that provided the data questioning the preventive role of fiber, a 1998 report showed that women who ate a diet high in red meat had higher rates of colorectal cancer. In that same study, women whose diets were low in red meat and high in fruits, vegetables, and cereal grains had a significantly decreased risk of colon cancer. In countries where diets are high in plant-based foods and low in red meat and animal fat, people have lower rates of heart disease and colon cancer.

Oatmeal has a high content of insoluble fiber which makes it an excellent food for your Power Diet-Step plan. Insoluble fiber helps shut off your appetite control mechanism because oatmeal is absorbed slowly from the intestinal tract. Oatmeal also has a high soluble fiber content, which helps to increase the good (HDL) cholesterol which in turn flushes out the bad (LDL) cholesterol from your bloodstream. Oatmeal and other high fiber bran cereals are also loaded with the mineral magnesium, which helps to regulate your insulin levels and reduces your risk of developing diabetes and obesity. Oatmeal for breakfast every day has been recommended by the American Heart Association as a great start for your day to reduce your risk of heart disease. People who eat oatmeal, as well as other whole-grain bran-type cereals daily, have less than one-half the risk of developing obesity and diabetes as non-cereal eaters. High-fiber bran cereals help to regulate insulin production in the morning. This helps to control your appetite and reduce the risk of gaining unwanted pounds. Oatmeal has also been shown to reduce your craving for high-refined sugar products and fatty foods.

FIBER KEEPS YOU HEALTHY

New findings from the Nurses' Health Study, reported in the *Journal of the American Medical Association,* showed that fiber, especially cereal products, protects against heart disease. This study examined the relationship between fiber consumption, as reported by nearly 70,000 women from 2014 through 2016. Women who ate an average of 30 grams of fiber a day had a 47% lower risk of major coronary events, including myocardial infarction and/or fatal coronary heart disease, compared to those who ate about half as much fiber. When the researchers analyzed the individual effects of three different fiber sources (fruits, vegetables, and cereals), only cereal fiber significantly reduced the risk of cardiovascular disease. A daily bowl of cold whole-grain breakfast cereal that supplies 5 or more grams of fiber cut heart disease risk by approximately 37%.

In this particular study of 70,000 women by the Nurses' Health Study, the ages of the women ranged from 37 to 64 years of age. None of the women in the study had a previous diagnosis of heart disease, stroke, cancer, diabetes, or high cholesterol. It is proposed that the increased consumption of whole-grain products may increase insulin sensitivity and lower triglyceride levels. Also, whole-grain products, including cereals, are important sources of phytoestrogens and may favorably affect blood coagulation activity.

The nutrients in fruits and vegetables, such as dietary fiber and antioxidants, are associated with a lower risk of heart disease, but few studies have examined their relationship to the risk for stroke. This study, reported in the *Journal of the American Medical Association*, described the association between fruit and vegetable intake and ischemic stroke in over 75,000 women enrolled in the Nurses' Health Study. Everyone in this particular study had no history of cardiovascular disease, stroke, cancer, diabetes, or high cholesterol. During the follow-up period, which included fourteen years for women, each increment of one serving of fruit or vegetables per day was associated with a 7% reduction for risk of ischemic stroke in women. This would translate into a *35% reduction in stroke for women* who ate five servings daily of fruit and vegetables. This study showed that there was no further reduction in the risk of stroke above 5-6 servings of fruit and vegetables per day. The consumption of a variety of vegetables and fruits, such as cruciferous vegetables (examples: broccoli and cabbage), green, leafy vegetables, citrus fruits or vitamin C-rich fruits and vegetables resulted in the largest decrease in risk. Pretty impressive results for sticking to your high-fiber colorful diet of fruits and veggies.

CHAPTER THREE RAPID READ

- Fiber blocks fat and burns calories for weight-loss, and also contains healthy ingredients that prevent many degenerative diseases, including heart disease, high blood pressure, strokes, and some forms of cancer.

- Fiber helps in weight loss and weight control because high-fiber foods contain **fewer calories for their large volume.** Fiber-rich foods are low in fat calories and have high water content. You are eating less and enjoying it more.

- High fiber foods have a **high bulk ratio**, which satisfies the hunger center more quickly than low fiber foods so fewer calories are consumed. Fiber-rich foods take longer to chew and digest than fiber-depleted foods, which gives your stomach time to feel full. Feeling full earlier leads to consuming fewer calories.

- Foods with **low-fiber content** are considerably **more concentrated in calories**.

- A high-fiber diet is essentially a **healthy, low-fat diet**, which decreases the intake of refined and processed food.

- High fiber good carbs **burn more calories during digestion** and make you feel fuller earlier **and longer** than eating refined bad carbs.

- Both fiber and protein help to curb your appetite by helping you to feel fuller earlier in the course of your meal.

- The consumption of a variety of vegetables and fruits, such as cruciferous vegetables (examples: broccoli and cabbage), green, leafy vegetables, citrus fruits or vitamin C-rich fruits decreases the risk for stroke and heart disease.

- Eating 30 grams of fiber each day is essential for weight loss.

FAT REALLY MAKES YOU FAT!

The typical American diet has a higher fat content than in nearly any other country in the world. There is little doubt that this increased fat intake in our diet is responsible for the development of obesity, as well as many other disorders. It is important to note that fat is the most concentrated source of calories, since a gram of dietary fat supplies your body with **9 calories**. This is compared to only 4 calories contained in each gram of protein or carbohydrate. Cutting down on the total fat intake is one of the best ways to cut down on the total number of calories, and to lose and maintain normal body weight.

It's very difficult to imagine how many fat calories that you consume each day. It's important to be able to find the fat in your diet and eliminate it. Everyone knows that there's fat in meat, sausage, bacon, lunchmeats, eggs, butter, ice cream, milk and cheese. But not everyone realizes that there's considerable fat in donuts, cakes, pies, muffins, margarine, mayonnaise, chicken and tuna salad, coffee creamers, yogurt, cream cheese, and cottage cheese. The more fat calories you consume, the more fat that will be stored in your body, and the more weight that you will gain. Dietary fat just fills up your fat cells because hardly any of the fat calories (only 5 out of 1,000) are used for digestion and are therefore not burned up. In other words, dietary fat not only is unhealthy, but it actually makes you fat.

Controlling our weight by reducing the amount of saturated fat in our diet has a two-fold benefit. First of all, it will help to control and maintain our weight. Secondly, it will have the beneficial effect of the prevention of cardiovascular and cerebrovascular disease (heart attacks and strokes), since these illnesses have been associated with high levels of blood cholesterol, which, in turn, come from the consumption of saturated fats.

Weight gain occurs from taking in more calories in the form of dietary fats than were burned off as fuel for energy. On a low-fat diet, calories are removed from storage in fat cells and are added to the fuel mixture of protein and carbohydrate for the production of energy. This results in permanent weight loss, unlike the temporary water weight loss of low-carbohydrate diets. Therefore, the less fat that you eat results in more storage fat being burned as fuel, and subsequently less fat is stored in your body. On the other hand, the more fat that you eat results in more fat being stored and less fat being burned, and consequently more fat cells remain in the form of fatty deposits throughout your body. The only way to lose even one pound of body weight is to burn approximately 3,500 calories. This can only be accomplished by cutting back on the total amount of fat in the diet, and also by increasing your physical activity. Nothing else works.

OBESITY: A RISK FACTOR FOR HEART DISEASE

In a study just released by the National Heart, Lung and Blood Institute in Bethesda, Maryland, obesity has now been listed as a major independent risk factor for heart disease. What's so new about that? Everyone knows that being overweight contributes to heart disease. That's just it; up until now obesity was just a contributing factor in heart disease because of its relationship with high blood pressure and high cholesterol. Now it has gained its own independent rating as causing heart disease all by itself. This study consisted of 3,500 women who were followed for 26 years. The risk of developing heart disease was more pronounced in women who gained most of their excess weight after the age of 25. In this study, obesity ranked fourth in women in predicting coronary heart disease. The other factors in heart disease were high blood pressure, serum cholesterol, cigarette smoking, age, diabetes and electrocardiogram abnormalities. Only high blood pressure, cholesterol and age were ranked ahead of obesity with cigarette smoking a close fourth in predicting heart disease. One important point made in this extensive study was that losing a moderate amount of weight lessened the risk of developing heart disease.

According to the American Heart Association in 2015 more than 41 million Americans have one or more forms of heart or blood vessel disease. **Heart attacks** claimed 650,000 lives, 56 percent of all deaths from cardiovascular disease. The Heart Association estimated that as many as one million Americans will have a heart attack this year and more than one-third of them will die.

FAT STORAGE IN WOMEN

In addition, the fat accumulated has to go someplace. You can see what's happening on the outside of you. Now, let's take a look at the inside. Fat infiltrates the liver and other organs. It's a squeeze process, an invasion. Fat compresses the heart, decreases the blood supply to the intestines and other organs. Some very obese people can't sit, because if they do, there's no space for their lungs to operate in, as the fat invades the chest. These people have to stand up or lie down all the time. They have disabled themselves. Along with all this, extra heavy people, and even moderately overweight persons, are putting an extra burden on their backs and legs (the weight-bearing joints), which causes or increases arthritic problems. Complications following surgery occur more frequently in obese people. Wounds don't heal as well or as fast. And again, since there is a breathing problem in obesity, overweight people can't take anesthesia as well as people of normal weight.

At a recent American Heart Association meeting, a study showed that men and women store fat in different places: men are more likely to store fat in their abdomens, whereas women store fat more easily in their buttocks and thighs, because nature gave women more fat cells there. What's the significance of these findings? Extra abdominal fat increases the risk of stroke, high blood pressure, diabetes and high cholesterol levels. The extra fat stored by women in the thighs and buttocks appear to be a harmless place to store fat according to this study; however, no woman wants to have fat thighs and buttocks. The good news is that women who walk seem to lose weight more easily in those trouble spots, making these areas firm and trim. Sedentary women can also store fat in their abdominal areas. So, no matter whether the fat is in your belly or in your buttocks, walking women stay slim and trim.

TYPES OF FATS

I. Saturated Fat

Saturated fat is present in all products of animal origin: meat, fish, fowl, eggs, butter, milk, cream and cheese. Saturated fats are also found in some vegetable products, which are usually solid or semi-solid at room temperature. They include shortenings and table spreads which have been changed from liquid fats (usually cottonseed and soybean oils) into solids by a process called hydrogenation. This process makes the products more suitable for table use and prevents them from becoming rancid. However, this process converts polyunsaturated fats into saturated fats. Other saturated fats in the vegetable kingdom include cocoa butter, palm oil and coconut oil. Most people are unaware of the fact that they consume significant amounts of coconut and palm oil. It is used commercially in a wide variety of processed foods, baked goods and deep-fat fried products.

Saturated fats are dangerous because they can increase the amount of cholesterol in the blood. These fats can raise the level of blood cholesterol as much as, if not more than, the actual consumption of dietary cholesterol products. These fats can also interfere with brain function and can actually cause damage to the brain cells by interfering with the brain's circulation. This can lead to memory loss, difficulty concentrating, and confusion and may even accelerate Alzheimer's disease. Saturated fats are also really bad fats and are solid by nature.

These fats raise your bad LDL cholesterol and lower your good HDL cholesterol. The DietWalk Plan on the other hand will lower your bad LDL cholesterol and increase your good HDL by following a low-fat diet and walking daily.

II. UNSATURATED FATS

1. **Monounsaturated fats** (neutral fats) may actually help to increase the good HDL cholesterol level, and, therefore, they have been found to be cardio-protective. These fats contain **omega-3 fatty acids**, which are extremely important in decreasing your risk of heart disease, degenerative diseases of aging and certain forms of cancer. They fats are usually liquid at room temperature and tend to harden or cloud when refrigerated. They are the primary fats found in olive oil, canola oil, peanut oil, most nuts and seeds, beans and lentils, avocados and some whole grain products.

   Fish oils. The fish oils contained in fish such as salmon, tuna, and haddock contain *omega-3 fatty acids*, have been recently found to improve exercise induced asthma. These omega-3 fatty acids appear to reduce the risk of heart disease, hypertension, strokes, blood clots, degenerative diseases of aging and some forms of cancer. Fatty fish are also low in total saturated fat and calories and satisfies your appetite easily due to its lean protein content. Poaching fish in water at a simmer (just below the boiling point of water) preserves the taste and texture of the fish. Any condiments can be added to the liquid to enhance the flavor, such as garlic or herbs.

2. **Polyunsaturated fats** (essential fatty acids) are always of vegetable origin and are liquid oils. Safflower oil is the highest in polyunsaturates of all oils. Sunflower oil is second, followed by corn oil, sesame seed oil, soybean oil, cottonseed oil, walnut oil and linseed oil. Polyunsaturated fats in limited amounts may help to lower the bad LDL cholesterol level by assisting the body to eliminate excessive amounts of newly manufactured

cholesterol. It is essential that you substitute monounsaturated and polyunsaturated fats for saturated fats to maximize their cholesterol-lowering effect. It is interesting to note that we can manufacture saturated fat and most monounsaturated fats in our bodies. Polyunsaturated fats, however, must be obtained from the diet and are, therefore, called *omega-6 essential fatty acids*. However, polyunsaturated vegetable oils, which are found in margarine, salad dressings, corn oil and processed foods, contain omega-6 fatty acids. These are also considered bad fats when excessive amounts are consumed, since they can set up chronic inflammation in brain tissue, which could lead to brain damage, strokes and degenerative brain diseases like Alzheimer's disease. Therefore, polyunsaturated oils should be limited to 1½ tsp. daily. Polyunsaturated fats are the good fats when eaten in moderation, but can turn bad when eaten in excess because of their omega-6 fatty acids that can cause inflammation in the body. Here we have an example of too much of a so-called **good fat.**

3. **Trans-fats** are fats that have hydrogen atoms added by either heat or pressure. They are formed when hydrogen atoms are added to oils containing mono or polyunsaturated fats. The hydrogenation process converts liquid oils into a more solid form. They then become hydrogenated (solid) or partially hydrogenated (semi-solid) oils and are **very bad fats.** They can increase your risk of heart disease by raising your bad LDL cholesterol and decreasing your good HDL cholesterol. They also have been reported to release a chemical called **Tumor Necrosis Factor**, which can cause inflammation in the body, thus increasing the risk for heart attacks, diabetes, high blood pressure and cancer. They are found in cooking oils, shortening, margarine many processed and baked foods, cookies, crackers, snack foods, and non-dairy creamers. Always check food labels for hydrogenated or partially hydrogenated oils, which are actually trans-fats.

Trans fats also cause you to gain more belly fat by redistributing stored fatty acids from various locations throughout the body and sending them into the abdominal fat cells. This increase in belly fat is thought to be due to the fact while trans fats cause a toxic reaction in the body's fat cells, causing them to discharge particles of fat globules into the bloodstream and relocating these fat globules into the abdominal area (the omentum which is a curtain of fat cells lining the abdominal intestinal organs). This omentum is located in the middle of the body and in the direct path of these traveling fat globules. Since there are so many fat cells located in the omentum, it is like a large fish net that catches all of these migrating fat cells and stores them as abdominal fat.

SAY NO TO YO-YO DIETS

The Framingham Heart Study, which has followed more than 5,000 people for almost 40 years, recently indicated a health hazard for chronic dieters. People who lost 10% of their body weight had an almost 20% reduction in the incidence of heart disease. So, what's the problem? These same dieters, who gained back the 10% of their body weight, raised their heart disease risk by almost 30%. So, if you weigh 160 lbs. and lost 10% or 16 lbs., you decreased your heart disease risk by 20%. But if you gained back that 16 lbs., you increased your risk of heart attack by 30%, an overall net gain of 10% and you still weigh the same 160 lbs. Sounds scary to me, folks! How many times have you heard the old saying that "I've lost enough weight over the years to equal two or three whole persons and I've gained every bit of it back?" Yo-yo dieting or weight-cycling makes it harder to permanently lose weight and is much more dangerous to your health.

Experts in the fields of physiology, biochemistry, psychology, nutrition and medicine have come up with the following startling findings about yo-yo dieting:

1. The **weight-loss/weight-gain cycle** actually increases your desire for fatty foods. Animal research studies at Yale University showed that rats that had lost weight rapidly on low-calorie

diets always chose more fat in their diets when given a choice between fat, protein, and carbohydrates. These rats always put on more weight than when they started the diet, and in a much shorter time than it had taken them to lose the weight.

2. **Yo-yo dieters increase the percentage of body fat** to lean body tissue with repeated bouts of weight gain and weight loss. People who lose weight rapidly on a low carbohydrate-high protein diet can lose a significant amount of muscle tissue. If the weight is regained again, they usually regain more fat and less muscle because it is easier for the body to gain fat than it is to rebuild muscle tissue.

3. **Body fat gets redistributed in the abdomen from the thighs, buttocks and hips** after weight cycling. Medical research has definitely shown that fat deposits above the waist increases the risk of heart disease and diabetes, not to mention an unsightly paunch.

4. When you lose weight by cutting calories, your *basal metabolic rate (BMR)* goes down, because it is the body's defense mechanism against starvation. The body can't tell the difference between starvation and low calorie dieting; consequently, your body is trying to conserve energy by burning fewer calories. This is the reason it becomes harder to lose weight after a week or two, even though you are eating exactly the same number of calories as you did when you first started your diet. This slow-down in the basal metabolic rate (BMR) persists even after the diet is over and accounts for the rapid-rebound, excessive weight gain that always happens to the dieter when she goes off her diet. This slow-down in metabolic rate can occur even after a single attempt at dieting. However, repeated effects of weight-cycling diets can affect the basal metabolic rate (BMR) much more, making additional weight-loss almost impossible and rebound weight gain almost inevitable. The yo-yo dieter is often heard to say, "I'm heavier now than I was before I started this damn diet."

5. An enzyme called *lipoprotein lipase (LPL)* becomes more active when you cut calories. This enzyme controls the amount of fat that is stored in your body's fat cells. Dieting, therefore, makes the body more efficient at storing fat, which is exactly the opposite of what a dieter wants. As you reduce your calorie intake, the enzyme LPL starts to activate the fat-storing process. This is another defense mechanism that the body uses to prevent starvation. Remember, the enzyme LPL doesn't know that you are dieting; it thinks that you are starving to death.

6. Women dieters who have lost a substantial amount of weight were compared to a group of normal weight people. After they lost weight, the previously obese individuals needed surprisingly fewer calories to maintain their weight than the normal-weight women. In this study, obese people who lost weight needed only 2000 calories a day to maintain their weight (125 lbs.) compared to 2300 calories per day to maintain the exact same weight (125 lbs.) by normal-weight people. Who said dieting was fair?

7. Chronic dieters who exhibited repeated cycles of weight gain and weight loss showed an increased risk of sudden death from heart attacks, according to a recent medical report. This study followed 1500 women over a period of 25 years who had engaged in cyclic-dieting.

SAY YES TO WALKING

We know that losing weight lowers blood pressure, reduces the risk of heart disease, lowers blood cholesterol and triglycerides and increases the HDL ("good" cholesterol). The answer is that dieting alone is not the best way to lose and maintain weight. The following is a list of the reasons why walking is the only safe and effective method to lose and maintain your ideal body weight:

1. **Exercise**, **particularly walking**, is the real answer to preventing the weight loss/weight-gain cycle from occurring. Walking makes it less likely you'll gain the weight back again because you

lose more fat and less muscle tissue with exercise. Also, walking prevents the slow-down in basal metabolic rate that always occurs with a yo-yo diet. Walking slightly **increases the BMR,** which helps to burn calories at a faster rate. Walking also **reduces the production of the enzyme *lipoprotein lipase (LPL)*,** which in turn decreases the amount of fat stored in the fat cells.

2. Walking also regulates the brain's appetite controller, the *appestat.* The more you walk, the more you decrease the appestat's hunger mechanism. Inactivity, on the other hand, stimulates the appetite control mechanism to make you hungry.

3. Walking, by increasing the aerobic metabolism of the body, **redirects the stomach's blood supply** to the exercising muscles, which in turn decreases your appetite.

4. And finally, walking encourages the body to *burn fat rather than carbohydrates*. This enables the body's blood sugar to stay at a relatively constant normal level. When the brain's blood sugar is normal we are not hungry. Both strenuous exercise and low-calorie dieting, however, burn carbohydrates rather than fats, causing a sharp drop in the blood sugar. When the brain's blood sugar drops as it does in low-calorie dieting or strenuous exercises, then we feel hungry in order to counteract this low blood sugar. The high fiber content of the DietWalk Plan also controls the body's appetite center, making overeating high-fat calories next to impossible.

POWER BREAKFAST WITHOUT THE FAT

Eating a healthy breakfast of complex carbohydrates (whole grain cereals and fruits) and lean protein (egg white, low fat milk or yogurt) combined with a morning walk will boost your metabolic rate all morning long after you have finished your breakfast and your walk. Skipping breakfast decreases your basal metabolic rate and leads to mid-morning snacking of refined sugars, (cakes, donuts, etc.) and coffee to feel your energy level boost.

Eating complex carbohydrates (fruits, vegetables, whole grain cereals, and nuts) uses up almost 25 calories out of every 1,000 calories consumed during the digestive process. So, it is quite evident that eating complex carbohydrates increases your post meal metabolic rate by burning more of the calories consumed during the digestive process. You are in effect burning some of the calories that you are eating rather than absorbing all of them into your body. A high fat, high carbohydrate breakfast (bacon, eggs, potatoes, and white bread) literally sticks to your ribs. Also, many types of granola cereals are usually high in fats and sugars and should be avoided as a breakfast cereal, unless their ingredients indicate that they are low in fat and sugar and have high fiber content (5 or more grams).

BOOST YOUR FAT-BURNING METABOLISM

1. You will burn more calories if you eat **small, frequent meals** or snack every three to four hours. Eating small, frequent meals help keep the body's **insulin level more even**, which makes it less likely you will store fat. If you go for a long period between large meals, your insulin levels spike, which makes it more likely you will store the extra calories and sugar as fat. This is because **sporadic surges in insulin levels** cause more sugar to be stored in your body's cells as fat, rather than being used as a source of fuel to produce energy.

2. People who eat a skimpy breakfast or no breakfast and very little lunch save up all of their calories for a big meal at dinner. This is probably the worst way to burn fat and the best way to store fat because of the inefficient utilization of glucose as a fuel. Instead **glucose gets turned into fat stores** in the body's cells.

3. If you eat every few hours you will have more energy because sugar will be used efficiently as **fuel to produce energy**. On the other hand, if you eat infrequently or wait until you are famished, then you will be fatigued because the sugar will not be able to be used as fuel efficiently, and energy production will go down.

a. Your brain needs **fuel to produce energy** to enable you to think clearly, concentrate, and to work efficiently. Also, your body needs fuel to help you exercise for longer periods of time, and to move faster and more efficiently. This steady supply of fuel can only be accomplished by a steady supply of glucose being utilized to produce the energy required for proper brain and body function.

b. **So the formula is:** small frequent, high fiber, lean protein, complex carbohydrate meals = steady level of insulin = constant supply of glucose = production of energy to boost body and mind functions.

4. It is important to have **a snack** (piece of fruit or a small amount of whole grain cereal) before your walking exercise workout (with or without weights), in order to increase your production of energy. Exercise stabilizes insulin and glucose levels, so that energy production is maximized. The combination of exercise and a small helpful snack improves your energy level.

5. On the DietWalk Plan, the addition of **lean protein** (lean meats, white meat of chicken or turkey, fish, non-fat dairy products including soy and egg whites, whole grains and bran, nuts, and seeds, all contribute to burning fat calories and boosting energy. Protein suppresses your appetite and produces the necessary fuel for the production of energy for all of your body's needs. Protein is made up of amino acids, which are essential for your cells' metabolism and for the repair and maintenance of all of your body's cells.

6. Several recent research studies have confirmed that people who consume two to three servings of **calcium containing foods** such as low-fat dairy products (milk, cheese, or yogurt) daily, lost considerably more weight than those individuals who just reduced their calorie intake, while consuming very little in the way of dairy products.

a. High calcium diets have been proven to inhibit the production of a certain calcium-regulating hormone, *calcitriol*, so that the amount of calcium and fat stored in the body's cells actually decreases. This actually causes you to store less fat, and ultimately lose more weight. On the other hand, it has been shown that low calcium diets actually increase this calcium-regulating hormone, which causes both calcium and fat to be stored in the body's cells and ultimately causes weight to be gained.

b. This calcium-regulating hormone works in conjunction with the protein found in dairy products to burn fat more efficiently and more quickly, which is another reason dairy products help you to lose weight. Research studies have also shown that low-fat dairy products have the same ability to limit fat storage and burn fat calories. So, non-fat milk, yogurt, and low-fat cheeses are ideal for a weight reduction program. For people who are lactose intolerant, lactose-free milk and yogurt work just as well.

MELT BELLY FAT

Refined carbohydrates that we eat are gradually absorbed into the bloodstream, which causes a sudden spike in insulin production. This excess amount of insulin in our blood causes these digested refined carbohydrates to head straight into our fat cells, particularly our belly fat cells, since the abdominal or belly fat cells are the closest to the digestive tract and contain the most concentrated amounts of fat cells in the entire body. Once the excess insulin has done its work by lowering blood sugar and packing fat into the fat cells of the abdomen, the low blood sugar which results in another round of carbohydrate cravings. It is like a "lose-lose combination."

As we age, we crave more carbohydrates, and the more carbs we eat, the more calories become stored as fat in our abdomen. Due to certain hormonal changes, which regulate our digestive system, we become less able to burn carbs for fuel, thus making carbs more likely to become stored as fat in the body, particularly in the abdomen. This actually becomes a vicious cycle since the more carbs we store as belly fat, the more carbohydrates we crave in our diet. Stored abdominal fat suppresses the formation of fat-burning hormones such as *leptin* which helps to keep blood sugars steady. Consequently, the more abdominal fat that you store makes it easier for you to gain more weight.

If you can diminish carbohydrate cravings, you'll subsequently lose unwanted belly fat. By eating high fiber foods, you can actually block the absorption of refined carbohydrates and starches. This is accomplished by increased fiber foods preventing the absorption of these refined carbohydrates by forming a web or net of fibers which encircles or tangles up these starches and carries them out of the digestive tract, almost completely intact and undigested. By blocking most of the absorption of these refined starches, less sugar and insulin are present in the bloodstream, which subsequently results in fewer cravings for carbohydrates. Less craving for carbs results in more belly fat being burned and more weight being lost, particularly around the abdomen.

High fiber foods, particularly beans (white, kidney, fava and pinto beans) contain an enzyme-blocking compound which blocks pancreatic enzymes (amylase and lipase) from breaking down refined starches. By inhibiting these enzymes from absorbing refined carbohydrates, your digestive tract bypasses absorption of these starches and transports them out of your digestive tract as though they were never totally digested. This results in a much slower rise in blood sugar, which in turn does not cause a spike in insulin production and consequently reduces your craving for carbohydrates.

BELLY FAT MELTING TIPS

THE FIBER-MINERAL COMBO—foods that contain both fiber and the mineral magnesium help to decrease the risk of developing the so-called **metabolic syndrome**. This syndrome consists of high blood pressure, diabetes, high blood fats, particularly triglycerides, insulin resistance, obesity and a tendency to accumulate excess amounts of abdominal fat. The combination of magnesium and fiber prevents sudden spikes in blood sugar and blood insulin levels that cause excess amounts of fat to become stored in your body's abdominal fat cells. Foods rich in magnesium include peas, beans (Lima and kidney beans), avocados, spinach, broccoli, whole grains, wheat germ, brown rice, sweet potatoes with skin and many fruits.

LOW-FAT DAIRY PRODUCTS (CHEESE, MILK, YO-GURT)—these low-fat dairy products suppress the hormone *calcitriol,* that causes fat to be stored in your abdominal fat cells. These low-fat dairy products also reduce the risk of developing the metabolic syndrome by up to 50%. Also, the combination of calcium and protein in these daily products combine to burn additional calories and help in weight-loss.

TRANS FATS—Avoid trans fats which can almost double your risk of developing abdominal fat deposits. These fats are either hydrogenated or partially hydrogenated oils that are found in margarine, fast and frozen foods, baked goods, non-dairy creamers and most packaged and processed foods. These fats can raise your blood pressure and increase your blood sugar, and therefore, block your arteries with cholesterol deposits. Recent research has shown that every 3 to 5% increase in the consumption of trans fats results in a 2-pound weight gain every four to six weeks, particularly around the abdominal wall.

AVOID STRESS—You can avoid stress by meditating, walking, doing yoga or any activity that you find calming. Stress unfortunately causes the body to produce the stress hormone *cortisol,* which can increase your blood fats, particularly triglycerides, and also increases your blood pressure and blood sugar. This deadly combination increases your risk of developing insulin resistance, which subsequently produces more belly fat, and thus increases the risk of developing the metabolic syndrome. Recent studies have shown that reducing cortisol production by engaging in calming activities and exercise helps to prevent the development of the metabolic syndrome with all of its attendant hazards, including excess storage of belly fat.

CHAPTER FOUR RAPID READ

- The only way to lose even one pound of body weight is to burn approximately 3,500 calories. This can only be accomplished by cutting back on the total amount of fat in the diet, and also by increasing your physical activity.

- Saturated fats are dangerous because they can increase the amount of cholesterol in the blood. Foods containing these include meat, fowl, eggs, butter, milk, cream, cheese and hydrogenated vegetable oils (often found in shortenings, table spreads, cottonseed and soybean oils).

- **Monounsaturated fats** (neutral fats) contain **omega-3 fatty acids**, which decrease the risk of heart disease, degenerative diseases of aging and certain forms of cancer. They are found in olive oil, canola oil, peanut oil, most nuts and seeds, beans and lentils, avocados and some whole grain products.

- The **weight-loss/weight-gain cycle** actually increases your desire for fatty foods. **Yo-yo dieters increase the percentage of body fat** to lean body tissue with repeated bouts of weight gain and weight loss.

- **Exercise, particularly walking**, is the real answer to preventing the weight loss/weight-gain cycle from occurring. Walking encourages the body to *burn fat rather than carbohydrates*.

- You will burn more calories if you eat **small, frequent meals** or snack every three to four hours.

- High-fiber foods prevent cravings for simple carbohydrates and will help reduce belly fat.

- Reducing stress and cortisol production by engaging in calming activities and exercise helps to prevent the development of the metabolic syndrome, which can lead to excess storage of belly fat.

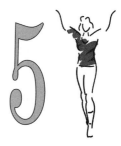

Dietwalk Weight-Loss Tips

WHAT TO THINK ABOUT BEFORE EATING

1. **Before food shopping, prepare a list and only go to the market after you've eaten.** Going to the market when hungry can lead to impulse purchases of high fat snack foods. Buy only those items on your list. Don't deviate from this list with snack foods, which you might have a tendency to buy, if you had not eaten prior to shopping.

2. When shopping for packaged or canned goods, **make sure the item of food you are purchasing has no more than 1.5—2.0 grams of total fat per serving.** If it is higher, compare other brands. Always look for non-fat or low-fat products; however, read the fat content on the nutritional label, and don't depend on a label that says "low-fat food." Many so-called low-fat items are fairly high in total fat content; for example, 2% milk has 5 grams of fat, and 98% fat free yogurt can have 3.5 to 4 grams of total fat. Always choose foods that are less than 2.0 grams of total fat. Also, watch out for labels that say "cholesterol-free." These foods may have 0 grams of cholesterol; however, they may contain many grams of total fat.

3. **Foods should be kept out of sight, in your refrigerator or pantry, between meals.** Do not place serving dishes on the table during meals to reduce the temptation to take second helpings.

4. **Don't skip meals.** Skipping meals lowers your blood sugar, which brings on cravings for high-carbohydrate, high calorie foods. Eating 3-4, or even 5, small meals per day is far better than eating one or two large meals. When your blood sugar remains constant, you are less likely to overeat.

5. **Eat meals more slowly.** Take smaller, less frequent bites and chew each mouthful for a longer period of time. Pause between each section of the meal. If you are still hungry when you are finished your first portion, wait at least 15 minutes to see whether or not you really want more. Leave the table as soon as you are finished eating and spend less time in the kitchen or areas that remind you of eating.

6. **Restrict your meals to one or two locations in your home for eating in order to avoid eating in every room.** This will reduce the tendency to snack during the day.

7. **Don't skip breakfast.** Individuals who skip breakfast usually wind up with a high fat, high-sugar snack mid-morning: the coffee break with a doughnut. A high fiber, low-fat cereal with fruit and skim milk will hold you comfortably until lunchtime.

8. **Don't use food as a stress reliever.** People have a tendency to seek out high-fat, high-sugar foods when under stress. Substitute music, reading, walking, meditation or a warm bath for food cravings.

9. **Don't start a weight reduction program just prior to the holiday season or before vacation time,** since these are the most unsuccessful times to begin a diet. The most important part of any successful diet is starting it. Once you've made up your mind to begin your diet, your half way there. You must be ready from the very beginning to discipline yourself. Just like every other part of your life, discipline is a must!

FOOD SELECTION AND PREPARATION

1. Eat salad greens and vegetables before the main course since these will take the edge off your hunger for higher calorie meat, poultry and fish portions. Substitute non-fat salad dressings or non-fat mayonnaise for regular varieties of these condiments. If not available, either use no dressing, or keep a small portion of dressing on the side and just dip your fork gently into the dressing every 2-3 bites of salad to get the taste without the added fat calories.

2. Soups and stews can be loaded with hidden fats. Refrigerate them overnight after preparing, and skim off the layer of fat that is lying on the surface of the stew or soup. This will remove more than 75% of the fat contained in these products. Choose soups loaded with vegetables and beans, and avoid any soups that are cream-based.

3. Hot foods, such as vegetable soups, and foods that require a lot of chewing will leave you with a greater feeling of satisfaction because they take a longer time to swallow and absorb.

4. Breads that are high in fiber, low in fat are the following: whole grain, bran-enriched, cracked wheat, whole-wheat pita, rye, pumpernickel and those labeled "high fiber breads." Avoid the high fat, low fiber breads: French, Italian, white, garlic bread, rolls and bagels. Remember to check the ingredients label. If the first ingredient doesn't say "whole," then it is not a whole-grain, high fiber bread. Choose whole wheat or oat bran English muffins, whole-wheat rolls or bread, whole wheat or oat bran bagels or raisin bread instead of sweet rolls, doughnuts, cakes and white bread. Remember to always scoop out the inside of rolls or bagels. Use jelly, honey, fruit preserves and all fruit jams, instead of margarine or butter, as spreads for your breads.

5. Make your meals attractive with colorful foods, garnishes and greens, such as carrots, tomatoes, broccoli, spinach, peppers,

yams, celery, and parsley, in order to make them more appealing. Also, vary your menu plans daily to avoid boredom. Remember that the more colorful the foods are, the more phytonutrients they contain.

6. Fresh vegetables and fruits are better choices than canned fruits and vegetables, which can be loaded with salt or sugar. Fruits and vegetable skins are excellent sources of fiber, as are the seeds, (berries, tomatoes, cucumbers, and pumpkins). Steamed vegetables, with or without herbs, can be cooked in a basket over boiling water. Steaming retains the flavor, color and nutrients of the vegetable.

7. Fresh or canned beans of any variety are excellent sources of fiber and vitamins. Their low-fat content makes them excellent companions to any meal. Make sure they are not prepared with meat (example: baked beans with bacon). Avoid high fat refried beans, but non-fat refried beans are okay.

8. Low fat, non-fat, or part skim-milk cheeses should be substituted for all other cheese. Make sure, however, that you check the total fat content per serving size. Non-fat yogurt is an excellent source of calcium and its lactobacillus, and other cultures are friendly bacteria for your colon.

9. Peeling a potato (white or sweet) before cooking or eating removes more than 25% of its nutrients and 35-40% of its fiber. A baked potato is an excellent food for meals or snacks (high fiber, low fat), compared to French fries, which are saturated with up to 15 grams of fat per serving. However, if you have a craving for French fries, you can prepare low-fat French fries by thinly slicing potatoes, spraying with non-fat vegetable spray, and baking for 20-30 minutes in an oven at approximately 300 degrees, or microwaving for 3 to 5 minutes. Keep your portion size small.

10. If you put salt on poultry, fish or meat before cooking, the food loses a good portion of its vitamin and mineral content during the cooking process. This is because the added salt causes the

food to be drained of its nutrients during the cooking process, which end up in the cooking broth.

11. Trim all visible skin and fat from poultry and meat before cooking. Either roast (using a rack), grill or broil meat, poultry and fish. The fat drips off during cooking. Baste with broth or vegetable juice to preserve moisture (defatted chicken broth is a good alternative). Or, a light dusting of olive oil is all that is necessary, and many companies now make olive oil sprays, which use considerably less fat than the tablespoon method. Never use butter, margarine, shortening, or gravy mixes.

12. Non-stick pans use less fat than cast iron, copper or aluminum pans. Use non-stick vegetable sprays as your first choice; otherwise, a small amount of olive oil (1 tsp.) or canola oil can be used for cooking.

14. Microwaving uses the foods' own moisture to cook. It's quick and easy, and you don't have to add any fat when microwaving. Almost all foods are microwaveable.

15. Stir-frying in a pan or wok is a fast way to make tasty vegetables, chicken, meats or fish. Add very small amounts of olive or peanut oil and seasonings followed by either defatted chicken broth or low-sodium soy sauce.

16. Sautéing: Use non-stick, non-fat vegetable sprays or a small amount of wine or defatted broth. Vegetables, fish, poultry or meats are mixed together in a pan. Then add herbs, such as thyme, basil, sage, or dill, for added taste.

17. Avoid sugary sodas, teas, juices and fruit drinks. Use fresh orange juice, grapefruit juice, tomato juice (low sodium), and non-caffeinated teas, coffee and diet sodas. Cream, whole milk, or powdered creamers should be avoided in coffee or tea; substitute skim milk or non-fat dairy creams. Avoid drinking a lot of artificially sweetened drinks as they can increase your appetite, due to the hypoglycemic effect (it lowers your blood sugar). But always make plain old water (tap or bottled) your drink of choice.

18. Non-fat milk has all of the calcium, vitamins and minerals that are present in 1%, 2%, or whole milk, and it tastes just as good. Non-fat milk or 1% milk, if that is preferred, in addition to building strong bones and muscles, has been shown to be effective in a weight loss program. Also, more recently, milk has been shown to contain certain anti-inflammatory fatty acids, which inhibit the formation of the COX-2 protein in the body. The COX-2 protein can cause inflammatory diseases such as cancer and arthritis. The fatty acids in milk exert an anti-inflammatory effect, which inhibits the formation of the COX-2 protein, and thus lessen inflammation in the body.

19. Coffee has a surprising number of health benefits. It contains an excellent source of antioxidants known as polyphenols. These plant compounds protect the body's cells from free-radical damage, which is responsible for a multitude of degenerative diseases. Coffee also improves mental acuity by enhancing cognitive performance and improving short-term memory. It also improves reaction time and enhances reasoning power, alertness, and attention span. The caffeine in coffee also serves as a wake-up call in the morning and also improves endurance during your daily activities. Coffee has been shown to have a number of positive benefits as long as you consume it in moderation and show no ill affects when you do drink coffee. Surprisingly, decaffeinated coffee also has a significant number of helpful antioxidants, which helps to prevent free-radical damage to your body's cells. Excessive amounts of caffeine, however, can cause irritability, nervousness, and insomnia in many people. Also, individuals with high blood pressure should avoid excess caffeine since it may aggravate existing hypertension.

20. Recent studies have shown that drinking cola products can actually elevate blood pressure considerably more than drinking coffee. Studies indicate that there are other substances in cola, besides just caffeine and sugar, which elevate the blood pressure considerably more than coffee does. Women who

drank large amounts of caffeinated cola beverages seem to develop high blood pressure. And surprisingly, the more coffee a woman drinks the less likely she was to develop hypertension. These findings were reported in a recent study in the Journal of the American Medical Association. Women who drank three or more cups of coffee per day had significantly less evidence of hypertension than women who drank three to four cans of cola whether it was sugared or sugar-free. Actually, the cola drinkers had a significant increased risk of developing hypertension compared to coffee drinkers who had very little evidence of hypertension.

SNACKS AND DESSERTS

1. A tasty non-fat dessert is angel food cake with fresh fruit and non-fat whipped cream. (A slice of cheese or chocolate cake has up to 14 grams of fat). The angel food cake, as described above, has less than 1.5 grams of fat.

2. Chocolate, particularly dark chocolate, contains healthful nutrients called flavonoids. These flavonoids are antioxidants that protect your heart from dangerous free radicals that can damage heart cells. These flavonoids also protect you from heart disease by decreasing the LDL bad cholesterol and increasing the HDL good cholesterol in the body. Chocolate also raises blood levels of endorphins (feeling-good hormones), which helps to relax you from anxiety and stress. Also, chocolate is actually good for a weight-loss program, because by just eating a small amount of dark chocolate, your appetite-control mechanism is quickly satisfied.

3. Sherbet, sorbet, frozen fruit bars and non-fat frozen yogurts are excellent substitutes for your ice cream sweet tooth.

4. Non-fat popcorn is an excellent low-fat, high fiber snack. Don't add butter or salt. Use hot air popper or microwave non-fat varieties.

5. Other low-fat snacks include hard pretzels (non-fat), soft pretzels (non-fat, SuperPretzel®), flavored rice cakes.

6. Excellent fat-free snack choices include dried or fresh fruits, raisins, peaches, apples, plums, apricots, bananas, baby carrots, and celery stalks.

7. Nuts are packed with nutrition and because of their protein content are very filling. They contain vitamin E, B-complex, folic acid, fiber, omega-3 fatty acids, and arginine (an amino acid). These nutrients contained in nuts have been shown to reduce bad LDL cholesterol and increase good HDL cholesterol and therefore help to reduce the incidence of heart disease and strokes. The nutrients in nuts also protect the heart against irregular heart rhythms and help to maintain your blood vessels' natural elasticity.

FISH: A GREAT DIET FOOD

Seafood is a good source of high-quality protein, nutrients and omega-3 fatty acids, which is an important part of a well-balanced healthful diet Also, fish is a great diet food since it's low in calories and saturated fat, high in protein and contains the heart-protecting, cancer-fighting benefits of omega-3 fatty acids. Even though shellfish has higher levels of cholesterol than other types of fish, it is low in saturated fat and therefore does not raise your blood cholesterol.

Fish are low in calories, low in fat, and high in protein, which makes them ideal for any real weight loss plan. Even shellfish with its higher content of cholesterol is still an important fat-burning food in your diet program. The low saturated fat content of shellfish offsets any cholesterol that these products may contain. The high protein content in fish acts as the fat-burner, since the protein increases your basal metabolic rate. Fat is subsequently burned more quickly and weight loss becomes quick and easy. Low mercury-containing fish eaten three times a week has been proven to help dieters lose weight easily and help to keep that weight off permanently. Fish also contain omega-3 fatty acids that help to reduce your risk of heart disease, strokes, cancer, and neurological disorders, such as Alzheimer's disease.

There is a type of fat contained in fish called omega-3 fatty acids, which is a form of polyunsaturated fats. These fats differ significantly from the omega-6 fatty acids, which are found in vegetable oil polyunsaturated fats. We are actually eating too many omega-6 fatty acids, which may counteract the good health benefits of the omega-3 fatty acids. To decrease your intake of omega-6's, avoid processed food snacks and baked goods made with cottonseed, sunflower, soybean, and safflower oils, especially those that say partially hydrogenated or hydrogenated oils, which are also high in the bad trans fats. Both olive and canola oils are low in omega-6 fatty acids. There are two types of omega-3 fatty acids. One is called DHA (*docosahexanoic acid*) and the other is EPA (*epicosapentaenoic acid*). These omega-3 fatty acids are found in cold-water fatty fish, such as salmon, tuna, mackerel, and sardines. They are also found in walnuts and flaxseed, which are plant sources of the omega-3 fatty acids.

EATING WHEN AWAY FROM HOME

Restaurant dining. The increase in obesity seems to coincide with the meals eaten out at restaurants, and not just fast-food restaurants. The portion sizes in restaurants are huge compared to the amount that you eat at home. Skip the French fries, fried foods, cheeseburgers, sodas, and high-fat dressings for salads. Always choose grilled or baked foods without breading. Order hardy vegetable soup whenever possible and avoid cream soups. And, most importantly, don't finish those oversized meals that most restaurants put in front of you, or you can order two appetizers instead of one large entrée. Eat one-half the meal and take the other half home, or share it with a friend. Otherwise, ask the waiter to wrap one-half of the meal before he brings it to the table, so that you don't eat more food than you really want to eat. Also, remember that when you're dining with friends or relatives, you're not obligated to keep up with the amount of food and drinks that they are consuming. Eat at your own pace and when you feel full, stop eating and wait until your companions are finished.

1. When eating out, choose low-fat foods without sauces, like broiled fish or chicken with a large tossed salad. Avoid alcohol, since it can increase your appetite and add extra calories. Incidentally, one gram of alcohol contains 9 calories, higher than a gram of fat, carbohydrate, or protein. If you like a drink with dinner, a wine spritzer is a good substitute, which is relatively low in total calorie value. Red wine (4 oz.) or a light beer every other night is also acceptable.

2. Don't be afraid to send back your meal in a restaurant if they didn't follow your order instructions. If you asked for steamed vegetables, baked potato, and broiled fish without butter, that's the way it should arrive on your plate.

3. At weddings and other parties choose the fresh vegetables and fruits without the dips. Avoid those fat-laden little appetizers with toothpicks in them. Consider the toothpicks red warning flags to stay away!

4. When traveling by air, order ahead for a low-fat meal when making reservations. They're available! Otherwise, if it is a short flight, have a low-fat snack prior to boarding.

5. Italian: Spaghetti or linguini is lower in fat than wider pastas that are often made with eggs. Try to order (when dining out) or buy whole grain pasta or spinach noodles for their high-fiber content. Stick to tomato or marinara sauces (however, some have too much oil, and you can have the waiter drain the oil from the pasta and bring back your dish). Seafood-based sauces without cream are also good substitutes.

6. Pizza can be ordered without cheese (tomato pie) and then add on a variety of fresh vegetables. If you want cheese, sprinkle on a little Parmesan cheese. Always blot off the extra fat on top of the pizza with a paper towel or napkin to absorb fat. By using this tip, you can remove more than 50% of the additional fat calories from the pizza.

7. Chinese restaurants: Stir-fry foods are better than deep-fried. Choose dishes with grains and vegetables. Order brown rice instead of white rice for the extra fiber content (not fried rice, which also comes out brown in color but is low in fiber). Ask to have your food prepared without soy sauce or MSG. Choose vegetable wonton soup or any vegetable-based soup rather than meat-based soups.

8. Mexican foods are great, if you can stay away from the deep-fried tortilla chips and order oven-baked chips with salsa instead. Skip the sour cream and guacamole (avocado), both of which are high in fat. Soft corn tortillas (tostadas or enchiladas) with chicken, tomato sauce and onions are good low-fat choices. Burritos or fajitas without sour cream or guacamole are excellent choices with lettuce, tomato and onion, and can be considered low-fat dishes. Avoid regular refried beans, deep-fried chimichangas, beef taco salad and deep-fried tortilla chips.

DIETWALK WEIGHT-LOSS TIPS

1. The most important part of the **DietWalk Plan** is to keep the **total fat content to no more than 30 grams daily** and to concentrate on heart-healthy fats and limit saturated fats. Not only does this accelerate your weight loss, but you decrease your risk of heart attacks and strokes by reducing your blood cholesterol levels.

2. An equally important factor in this diet is the **30 grams of dietary fiber** that you will be eating every day. Since fiber is primarily plant based, you will be eating lots of soluble and insoluble fiber, which also helps to reduce your cholesterol in addition to reducing your appetite. These high fiber plants also contain numerous beneficial compounds including phytonutrients, antioxidants, flavinoids, B & C vitamins, minerals, beta and other carotenoids and folic acid, among others. All of these compounds help to fight heart disease, cancer, and many other degenerative diseases.

3. Remember to **eliminate all refined foods** (sugar, flour and rice) and **packaged and processed foods** and commercially **baked goods.** Also, limit the amount of **salt** (which can cause fluid retention and can lead to hypertension), **caffeine** (which can stimulate your appetite and cause anxiety, palpitations, and even high blood pressure) and alcohol (which adds additional calories to your diet); limit alcoholic drinks (3-4 ounces red wine or 12 ounces light beer) to 3 to 4 times per week.

4. Enjoy at least **2-3 servings from the fruit group and 2-3 servings from the vegetable group** each day which helps to control your appetite on the DietWalk plan. For a wide variety of nutrients, choose fruits and vegetables in a rainbow of colors. In most cases within reason, you can *eat as many fresh fruits and vegetables (raw or steamed—no butter or oils added) as you'd like to eat.*

5. Choose from an array of **high-fiber, nutritious, complex carbohydrates** that fill you up without filling you out. These foods provide high-octane fuel to power you through the day and keep you energized for physical activity. The following foods are excellent sources of fiber: barley, oats, bran, wheat germ, bulgur and brown rice; beans, peas and lentils; wholegrain breads and pastas; and most fruits and vegetables (see Fat & Fiber Counter in Chapter 10). Remember, the increased intake of fiber is what keeps the DietWalk plan working. In other words, the more fiber you eat, the less weight you'll gain. *Fiber fills you up without making you fat.*

6. Make sure your diet contains adequate **lean protein,** which is essential for proper nutrition and metabolism. Protein helps to heal, repair and maintain all of your body's cells and to regulate your basal metabolic rate. Some good sources of lean protein are egg whites; low or non-fat dairy products such as cheese, milk, yogurt and soy products; nuts, seeds and beans; very lean meats, white meat of chicken or turkey without the skin, fish; and whole grain cereals, breads and pastas.

7. **Drink at least six 8 oz. glasses of water daily.** Water fills you up so that your appetite is decreased, especially if you drink 8 oz. of water before your meals.

8. **Be careful of soft drinks.** Sweetened soft drinks contain loads of sugar and calories. These include: sodas, sweetened iced teas, fat-laden calories in coffee drinks such as lattes and cappuccinos, and juices that contain little or no juice, but lots of sugar. Stay away from the so-called energy drinks, which contain high amounts of sugar and caffeine. These drinks are unhealthy and the energy that they produce initially is from the initial shot of caffeine and glucose absorbed into the bloodstream. These drinks cause unhealthy spikes in both blood sugar and blood insulin, and the high caffeine content of these drinks can be dehydrating. Choose low sugar sodas and teas without artificial sweeteners. Switch to fat-free coffee drinks without sugar. Choose 100% fruit juices and 100% vegetable juices. Drink lots of water, seltzer, and fat-free milk.

9. **Limit the amount of salt, caffeine, and alcohol** in your diet. Excess amounts of salt and caffeine in your diet can raise your blood pressure and cause heart rhythm abnormalities. Both salt and caffeine can actually increase your appetite. Excessive alcohol intake can add unwanted calories to your diet (9 calories per gram) and could possibly damage your liver. However, several medical studies have shown that 4 ounces of red wine daily can be a heart-healthy addition to your diet, since it contains a powerful antioxidant called *resveratrol.*

10. **Always check the labels when buying food.** See how many calories are in a serving size and also check how many servings are in the entire package that you are considering purchasing. Make sure that the saturated fat and the sugar contents are low. The first listed ingredient on the ingredients label is the one that contains the highest concentration in the food that you are buying. If sugars or fats are listed first, then put it back on the shelf.

11. **Portion control** is the key to any successful diet. Serve your meals on small plates to limit the amount that you eat. Eat slowly and stop when you feel full, no matter how much food is left on the plate. Remember, that you don't have to finish everything on your plate. In order to lose weight, you must eat less food. People have a tendency to clean their plates, no matter how large the portion size is. Avoid oversized bowls and plates at home, which hold larger portions. Concentrate on smaller servings and pause during a meal to give your appetite control mechanism time to let you know that you're actually full. Be careful not to eat fast, because you will consume mass quantities of calories before you'll ever know that you're not hungry any longer.

12. **Vitamin D,** either in supplement form or manufactured in your body by exposure to the sun, appears to reduce the risk of certain forms of cancer, particularly prostate cancer. The active ingredient in vitamin D is *calcitrol*, which appears to slow or inhibit the growth of cancer cells. If you are not able to have sun exposure, particularly in the winter, then the recommended daily allowance is 200 IU (ages 20-50); 400 IU (ages 51-70); and 600 IU (over the age of 70).

13. Three-four ounces of **red wine** every other day is heart healthy since the red grapes contain *resveratrol*, a super antioxidant which helps to prevent strokes, blood clots, hypertension and heart disease, this providing that you have no underlying liver or cardiac problems which prevents consumption of any alcoholic beverages. You can get the same benefits by eating red grapes or purple grape juice without the alcohol.

14. **High protein** foods appears to have a blood pressure lowering effect, particularly when consuming vegetable protein rather than meat protein. Also, the unique combination of protein and calcium in non-fat or low fat dairy products helps to keep your appetite satisfied for a relatively long period of time. Also, this calcium and protein combination found in dairy products appears to increase the metabolic rate and burn fat calories faster.

15. **Food cravings** are a constant battle in the war against overeating. When you're under stress or anxious, you have a tendency to crave high calorie foods and sweets. You can overcome food cravings by eating low calorie, crunchy foods such as celery, carrots, apples, rice cakes, popcorn, nuts, seeds and low fat pretzels. The crunch factor helps to reduce stress and anxiety by relaxing your tense neck and facial muscles. Fruits are also a great way to combat sweet food cravings. Also, lean protein and low fat products, high fiber foods produce good-feeling hormones (endorphins and serotonin), which helps to prevent you from giving in to food cravings for sweets and high fat foods.

16. **Calcium burns fat calories.** Several new studies have shown that people who regularly drink skim milk and eat yogurt or have one serving of cheese per day lose an average of 1½ pounds per month, with no additional change in their diets. It is believed that calcium decreases the stores of fat in the fat cells by actually burning stored fat. Also, it is thought that the protein content in milk, yogurt and cheese replaces the fat stored in the fat cells by a unique process of providing extra protein to the body's cells. This combination of calcium and protein which is present in milk, yogurt, and cheese helps the body to burn fat and store protein. A study at the University of Tennessee suggests that calcium found in these foods actually blocks fat storage in the cells that plump up your abdomen, thighs and hips. This calcium also has the added advantage of increasing your good HDL cholesterol and decreasing your bad LDL cholesterol. Non-fat milk and low-fat cheeses and non-fat or low-fat yogurts have the same amount of minerals, vitamins, protein and calcium as whole milk without the added fat content. And, as far as your diet is concerned, fat-free milk contains only 80 calories per glass and is packed with 220 mg. of calcium.

You can lose up to 12 lbs. in only 2 weeks, and re-shape your body, as you easily get rid of those unwanted pounds. It is likely that your weight-loss will taper-off very slightly after the first 14 days;

however, you will still be able to lose approximately 3-4 pounds every week as your body's metabolism adjusts to the DietWalk weight-loss plan. The weight you lose will stay lost forever.

CALORIES DON'T COUNT! YES, THEY DO!

According to a recent study in the *Journal of the American Medical Association*, there is a no magic formula to losing weight. You can lose weight by following a variety of different diet programs; however, the one thing that always counts is the number of calories that you consume vs. the number of calories that you burn daily.

Yes, even those horrendous, low-carbohydrate diets also work; however, that's because they restrict calories also, not just carbohydrates. Also, they work because you are creating an unhealthy condition found in diabetics called ketosis, where you are burning protein instead of fat to lose weight. Unfortunately, the weight comes back twice as fast when you stop the diet, if, however, you are fortunate enough not to have damaged your liver or kidneys while you were on this stupid diet.

Unfortunately, Americans have been gaining so much weight in the last twenty years that obesity is becoming an actual epidemic. Over 60% of adults are overweight, including approximately 30% who are considered obese. This trend has almost tripled in teenagers during this same time period.

After reviewing over 100 diet studies since 1966, researchers concluded that if you want to lose weight, you should consume fewer calories daily over a long period of time. By restricting one type of food over another, as in the low-carbohydrate diets or high-protein diets, you are making a weight loss program more difficult, and more dangerous.

A low-fat, high-fiber diet with moderate amounts of vegetable protein and complex carbohydrates is the single, best healthy weight loss diet that you can follow for good health and permanent weight loss. There are no dangerous side effects, no feelings of hunger, and you have the added benefit of a diet that is actually good for you. You will have less weight, less heart disease and hypertension, less strokes and dementia, and a lower incidence of several forms of cancer. This diet, by its very nature, turns out to be a low-calorie diet in disguise, and what's more, it actually works and keeps on working. The DIET-WALK plan is a healthy diet that you can follow for a lifetime to lose and maintain your ideal weight, and maintain good health, longevity, and physical fitness.

FOOD JOURNAL

It is important to keep track of when and what you eat at each and every meal, including snacks. It is just as important to be conscious of why you eat, especially when you are nibbling snacks unconsciously throughout the day, or eating more calories than you should consume at meal time. Were you watching TV and not paying attention to what you were eating? Were you in a meeting or at work or talking on the phone and eating junk food without really noticing what you were eating?

A food journal can help you solve these problem areas by keeping an accurate record of what you actually eat at each and every meal on each and every day. This record will enable you to establish a more realistic diet plan as you move forward on your Power Diet-Step weight loss plan.

You can keep your record of your food diary in a notebook or you can do it online at www.myfooddiary.com. To count the total number of calories and the number of grams of fat that you consume at each meal, you can consult any one of a number of food nutrition books, or you can go to any of the websites that list the calories of different foods and also lists the number of grams of carbohydrate, protein, and fat for each food. One such website is www.calorielab.com.

When you combine the DietWalk: 30 Grams Fat / 30 Grams Fiber Plan with 30 Minutes of walking you have the ideal weight loss plan. When you start to formulate your own meal combinations of 30 grams fat/30 grams fiber, you should keep a **daily record of the total grams of fat and the total grams of fiber** that you eat at each meal. Make sure that the total for each day adds up to no more than 30 grams of total fat and no less than 30 grams of fiber. You can use 3 x 5 index cards to keep your record for each individual meal. After you've recorded your meals each day, store the cards in a 3 x 5 index box divided into 4 sections: breakfast, lunch, supper, and snacks. Then you can thumb through your cards at a later date to look up any meal that you'd like to have without having to add up the fat and fiber grams again. Or record your meal plans on your computer or on any hand-held electronic device or smart phone. Choose any method that's easy, convenient and fun for you. You will lose weight quickly and easily on the *DietWalk Plan* without worrying about rebound weight gain.

A food journal gives you a basic guideline of what you have been doing wrong and the means to correct your food eating habits. Make sure that you record everything that you consumed in any given 24-hour period.

QUICK TIPS FOR WATCHING WEIGHT

1. Drink one cup of fat-free milk instead of one cup of whole milk. Add nonfat milk to your coffee, cappuccino, or lattes.

2. Use 1 tablespoon of mustard, ketchup, or fat-free mayonnaise instead of regular mayonnaise in salads or on sandwiches. Mix ketchup and nonfat mayonnaise to make a delicious Russian dressing. Served on a wedge of iceberg lettuce, it makes a tasty snack.

3. Share a small bag of potato chips or French fries with a friend, or skip them altogether, or just taste three or four and throw the bag away.

4. Cut a slice of pizza in half and save the other half for later in the day.

5. Check serving sizes of your favorite foods when you eat out. For example:

   a. One-half cup of cooked cereal or pasta at home is equivalent to a single serving size; however, restaurant portions are equivalent to approximately three serving sizes, and that's before they even add the sauce.

   b. One-half of a bagel is one serving, but a deli bagel is equivalent to at least three servings.

   c. One small pancake or waffle at home is equal to one serving size, but in a restaurant, one pancake is about two and one-half servings.

d. A dozen potato chips or tortilla chips equal approximately one serving; however, a small bag contains at least two to three servings.

6 Always check the serving sizes on any prepackaged food that you get. Most people, when they consume a package of processed foods, assume that it is one serving size, when it may be two to three serving sizes.

Be careful of prepackaged foods that contain trans fats. Trans fats are identified as partially hydrogenated oils. They are not listed or labeled on the package as trans fats. The FDA will be requiring foods to have trans fats listed, but that won't occur until 2006. The reason trans fats are dangerous is that they raise the blood levels of cholesterol and saturated fats and lead to heart disease, hypertension, and strokes.

A DRINK FOR HEALTH AND BEAUTY

Most people don't realize that they don't drink enough water. Recent studies have indicated that at least ¾ of adults walk around chronically dehydrated, because they forget for one reason or another to drink a recommended six to eight 8-ounce glasses of water daily. A chronic dehydration can lead to kidney damage, dizziness, headaches, and irregular heart rhythms, particularly palpitations.

Adequate water consumption is necessary for all the body's metabolic functions and for the health of all of the body's organs, tissues, and cells. Water is essential for digestion, kidney function, respiratory and cardiac health, and the metabolism of the entire body. Without adequate water intake, you run the risk of many health disorders. One way to keep regularly hydrated is to make sure that you drink water before, during, and after each meal. If you drink just 4 ounces of water at a time frequently throughout the day, you can trick yourself into drinking the recommended six to eight ounces of water daily. Also, water fills you up without filling you out and helps to decrease your appetite so you consume fewer calories. Here you have an easy weight loss drink. Dieters who sip water all day tend to lose more weight than people who drink less water daily. Drinking water has a significant effect on a dieter's success, since water has no calories and reduces food cravings; it controls your appetite by making you feel full with a zero-calorie drink.

Surprisingly, water increases the flow of blood to your skin and gives your face a rosy glow by dilating small skin capillaries when you are well-hydrated. Also, good hydration is helpful in providing an increased flow of blood to all of your body's cells, which improves your metabolism at a cellular level. When you are well hydrated, you will lose weight, feel great, and look younger.

Water also helps to prevent kidney stones by diluting substances in the blood like calcium and then flushes these diluted substances out of the body. New studies suggest that water also reduces the intensity and duration of migraine headaches. This is apparently due to an increased blood supply to the brain. And lastly, water has been shown to reduce the incidence of colds and flu-like viruses by hydrating the membranes of the nasal and throat passages, making it difficult for viruses to embed themselves in or on dry mucous membranes.

Whether your exercise is indoors or outside, if you exercise strenuously, your body can become depleted of both water and potassium. Make sure that you eat a banana or piece of fruit when you exercise. Water rehydrates your body and bananas supply the mineral potassium that was depleted from your exercise. Recent research has found that even those individuals who engage in moderate types of exercises need to be rehydrated with water and potassium after their exercise. Potassium is the mineral that works with mineral sodium to balance the fluids and electrolytes in your body. The main function of potassium is to maintain the electrolyte and fluid balance in your body. Potassium regulates your heartbeat and prevents muscle cramping and muscle fatigue.

WEIGHT-LOSS MYTHS

Myth No. 1—The more you perspire, the more calories you burn, and the more weight you lose.

This is a myth because some people just perspire more than others do. Extra sweating doesn't mean that you're burning extra calories. The key to burning more calories and losing more weight is twofold. One, it's the intensity of your workout that determines how many calories you burn. If you're breathing hard and your muscles feel sore, then you're burning extra calories. Secondly, and actually more importantly, is the duration of your exercise. Moderate, low-intensity exercises, like walking for 30 to 45 minutes, burn more calories than short-term strenuous exercises without the muscle aches or the heavy breathing. By increasing the basal metabolic rate for a longer period of time, the body burns calories at a steady rate while exercising, and even continues to burn calories at a lower rate after the exercise is finished. This is because the basal metabolic rate doesn't slow down immediately after your longer duration moderate exercise. Moderate, steady exercise, like walking, again wins the fitness race.

Myth No. 2—Lifting heavy weights either on machines or free weights, burns more calories than lifting light to moderate weights.

Lifting heavy weights does burn more calories initially; however, since this activity cannot be continued for a long time, calories are only burned short-term. Besides, heavy weight lifting is essentially unhealthy, since it can cause muscle and ligament tears and various other tendon injuries. Interestingly enough, studies have shown that lifting heavy weights may contribute to the development of high blood pressure, since this is an anaerobic exercise, which does not produce oxygenation of all of the body's cells, like aerobic exercises do.

Strength-training exercises, using light to moderate weights, can be continued for a longer duration, which leads to the steady burning of calories. It actually boosts your overall metabolism. This leads to weight loss and the gradual sculpting of muscles for a better, not bigger, figure. Also, these strength-training exercises help to prevent thinning of the bones as we age (osteoporosis). These exercises build more muscle, which burns more calories than fat, even after you stop exercising. Again, we have an example of slow and steady wins the fitness and weight-reducing race. And in this particular case, the muscle and figure-improving race.

***Myth No. 3*—A morning workout like running burns more calories than at any other time of day, and subsequently you will lose more weight quickly.**

Calories burned are dependent on the type and duration of exercise that you do. It has nothing to do with the time of day. Your body can't differentiate between a morning or an evening workout. All that your body knows is how many calories you've burned by the duration and the type of exercise you are doing at any particular time of day. The same formula holds, no matter when you exercise. It takes burning 3500 calories to lose one pound of body fat. This can take a day, or a week, or a month; the calories that are burned are cumulative. In other words, if you burn 350 calories a day walking, you will lose a pound of body fat in ten days (350 calories x 10 days = 3500 calories burned).

***Myth No. 4*—Anything that you eat in the evening will turn to fat, since you're inactive in the evening and while you're sleeping.**

This is another myth regarding weight loss. It doesn't make any difference when you eat. It's the total number of calories that you consume daily vs. the total number of calories that you burn daily that determines weight loss or weight gain. Your body does not differentiate calories eaten during the day or in the evening, only how many calories you have eaten on that particular day. The only disadvantage to eating late in the evening is if you have a condition known as reflux, and in that particular case, this could precipitate heartburn. If you do have reflux, it is certainly essential to have this checked by your physician.

Myth No. 5—**Running and strenuous aerobic exercises are the best way to lose weight.**

Strenuous exercises burn primarily carbohydrates during the first two-thirds of your workout, and then begin to burn fat only during the last one-third of the workout. Walking and moderate exercises, on the other hand, burn fat during the first two-thirds of your workout, and then burn carbohydrates in the last third of the workout. You can clearly see that you will burn more calories (fat has 9 calories per gram compared with carbohydrates, which have 4 calories per gram) by moderate exercises like walking.

Strenuous exercises are not only ineffective in a weight-reduction program, but they are dangerous, since they contribute to muscle and ligament injuries, strains and sprains, and have even been known to cause more serious problems like heart attacks and strokes.

A recent study from the University of Pittsburgh found that women who rated their exercise as moderate lost a comparable amount of weight, if not more weight, than those women who exercised vigorously. It's the total duration of activity, and not the intensity of activity, that burns more calories. Weight loss occurs more gradually and more effectively in a moderate exercise program like walking. Walking also contributes to the maintenance of weight loss for as long as you continue your walking program.

Myth No. 6—**Fasting for one or two days can help you to lose weight.**

On the contrary, fasting does not lead to weight loss, because your body metabolism slows down considerably. The body is attempting to conserve calories, since it thinks that you are starving to death, and wants to prevent you from getting sick. So, calories are burned at a much slower rate and it's unlikely you will lose any weight at all by fasting. Besides, once you resume your food intake, your body's metabolism remains in its slow-down phase until it's sure that you're not starving. During this time, most of the calories you eat get stored in fat cells and you are likely to gain extra weight instead of losing weight.

Myth No. 7—**Vegetarian diets are healthier and help you lose weight more easily than non-vegetarian diets.**

Again, it's the total number of calories consumed daily that determines weight loss or weight gain. This occurs regardless of whether you are eating vegetables or meat. The only problem with a strict vegetarian diet that doesn't allow meat, fish, fowl, or dairy is that you are losing essential vitamins and minerals that your body needs. You must supplement these losses with a multivitamin and mineral supplement. Also, strict vegetarians can become protein-deficient and have to rely on nuts, legumes, and soy for their protein. Strict vegetarians also tend to consume many refined carbohydrate, processed foods, which are high in fat and calories. So, it's unlikely that a strict vegetarian diet is better for weight loss than a more balanced, low-calorie, low-fat, moderate protein and complex carbohydrate-type of diet.

CHAPTER FIVE RAPID READ

- Foods should be kept out of sight, in your refrigerator or pantry, between meals.
- Don't skip meals.
- Eat meals more slowly.
- Restrict your meals to one or two locations in the home for eating to avoid eating in every room.
- Don't use food as a stress reliever.
- Don't start a weight reduction program just prior to the holiday season or before a vacation.

Food Selection and Preparation:

- Before food shopping, prepare a list and only go to the market after you've eaten.
- Make sure the item of food you are purchasing has no more than 1.5-2.0 grams of total fat per serving.
- Eat salad greens and vegetables before the main course to take the edge off your hunger for higher calorie portions.
- Hot foods and foods that require a lot of chewing will leave you with a greater feeling of satisfaction.
- Vary your menu plans daily to avoid boredom. A low-fat, high-fiber diet with moderate amounts of vegetable protein and complex carbohydrates is the single, best healthy weight loss diet that you can follow for good health and permanent weight loss.
- It is important to keep track of when and what you eat at each and every meal, including snacks.
- Water is essential for digestion, kidney function, respiratory and cardiac health, and the metabolism of the entire body. Make sure that you drink water before, during, and after each meal.

- When eating out, choose low-fat foods without sauces, like broiled fish or chicken with a large tossed salad.

- A low-fat, high-fiber diet with moderate amounts of vegetable protein and complex carbohydrates is the single, best healthy weight loss diet that you can follow for good health and permanent weight loss.

- It is important to keep track of when and what you eat at each meal, including snacks. A food journal can give you a basic guideline of what you have been doing wrong and how to correct your food eating habits.

- Check serving sizes of your favorite foods when you eat out or on prepackaged foods.

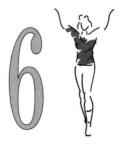

WALKING WOMEN WIN!

YES, WOMEN ARE DIFFERENT FROM MEN!

"Yes, Women *ARE* Different From Men" was the first page headline in *The Medical Tribune*. New research has discovered that there are significant differences in the physiology of women and men. These differences extend far beyond the obvious reproductive biology differences. These differences affect almost every organ system in the body, including the heart, brain, digestive tract, nervous system, and even the skin.

With reference to the heart, women's hearts beat faster at rest than do men's hearts. Also, the electrical behavior of the conducting tissue in the heart is different in women and men, which may explain the normal difference in the EKGs of women and men. It has previously been found that a woman's coronary arteries are smaller than those of a man. These factors have to be taken into consideration in the diagnosis, treatment, and prevention of heart disease in women. Physicians are just recognizing the difference in treating women with coronary artery disease.

Men's brains are larger than women's brains; however, women's brains contain more neurons (nerve connections), which may explain why women are better at multi-tasking (juggling more things simultaneously in their lives—work, child care, home responsibilities, social activities, and caring for their big-brained mates). Face it, women are different from men, and smarter, too.

A long-held fallacy in medicine has been that whatever research was done on male patients—for example, physiology and reactions to different medications—could be interpreted as being the same for women. Nothing could be farther from the truth. For example, women metabolize different medications differently from men, which must be taken into careful consideration when treating female patients. Many diseases and medications affect women differently and these differences must be recognized when formulating different types of treatments for various diseases. Yes, women are really different from men, and it's about time that the medical establishment is becoming aware of that important difference.

Many of these differences in physiology may explain the difference in the fitness response to exercise in women. The *maximum oxygen uptake* is defined as the highest rate at which oxygen can be taken up from the atmosphere and utilized by the body during exercise. It is frequently used to indicate the cardio-respiratory fitness of an individual. Even though men have a larger overall muscle mass than women, women have more long-term endurance capacity. This may in part be explained by a woman's ability to sustain her maximum oxygen uptake longer by steady, consistent exercise.

Men frequently engage in short bursts of energy expenditure like jogging, racquetball, strenuous weight lifting, etc. This type of strenuous activity does not increase the maximum uptake capacity (uptake and distribution of oxygen throughout the body) for a long enough time to develop maximum aerobic fitness. Women, on the other hand, develop aerobic fitness more slowly than men; however, their fitness and endurance levels are more consistent and long lasting. In other words, women who engage in moderate exercise activity like walking, stationary bike, treadmill, etc., are more likely to stay aerobically fit than men.

WHY WALK?

The second component of the DIETWALK Plan is the *30 minutes of aerobic walking 6 days per week;* The aerobic walking program for 30 minutes causes your body's metabolism to burn calories during and also after you're walking. You'll be surprised how good you feel after your 30-minute walk, with increased energy and vigor. The additional flow of oxygen throughout your bloodstream will increase your metabolic rate, so that you will burn calories more quickly. This increase in metabolism will allow you to lose weight more quickly and will improve your cardiovascular fitness.

With the advent of the computer age, women are forced by design to do less and less physical labor. It would seem logical that this would result in more energy being available for other activities. However, how many times have you noticed that the less you do, the more tired you feel, whereas the more active you are, the more energy you have for other activities? Exercise improves the efficiency of the lungs, the heart, and the circulatory system in their ability to take in and deliver oxygen throughout the entire body. This oxygen is the catalyst that burns the fuel (food) we take in to produce energy. Consequently, the more oxygen we take in, the more energy we have for all of our activities.

Oxygen is the vital ingredient that is necessary for our survival. Since oxygen can't be stored, our cells need a continuous supply in order to remain healthy. Walking increases your body's ability to extract oxygen from the air, so increased amounts of oxygen are available for every organ, tissue, and cell in the body. Walking actually increases the total volume of blood, making more red blood cells available to carry oxygen and nutrition to the tissues, and to remove carbon dioxide and waste products from the body's cells. This increased saturation of the tissues with oxygen is also aided by the opening of small blood vessels, which is another direct result of walking.

So, let's take that first step for energy, fitness, and pep. Walking every day will keep a fresh supply of oxygen surging through your blood vessels to all of your body's hungry cells. Don't disappoint these little fellows because you depend on them as much as they depend on you.

If you short-change them on their daily oxygen supply, they'll take it out on you in the form of illness and disease. A 30-minute walk a day keeps the doctor away.

The basal metabolic rate, like the energizer bunny, keeps on ticking even after you have stopped walking. Your body's normal resting basal metabolic rate burns approximately one calorie per minute (CPM). During your regular 30-minute daily walk at 3.5 miles per hour, your basal metabolic rate increases to five calories per minute. Now, here is the so-called "slight-of-hand-walking-trick." When you stop walking your basal metabolic rate does not return to its resting one calorie per minute rate. Your body's metabolic rate got so revved up from your 30-minute walk it continues to remain elevated for up to six hours after you have stopped walking. This increased rate will not remain at five calories per minute, but it will stay at between two to three calories per minute for the next six hours. What does all that mean? Well, if you walk for one half hour during lunch, when you get back to the office and are stuck behind your computer for the rest of the day, your body's metabolic rate will be burning two to three calories per minute instead of the usual sedentary one calorie per minute if you had not walked at lunch time. The same process will occur if you take a one-half hour walk after supper. You will actually be burning an additional two to three calories per minute while you are sleeping rather than the resting one calorie per minute metabolic rate. This actually means that you will burn more calories everyday while you walk and at rest after you walk.

In effect, you have discovered a double blast of calorie burning. One with exercise and one with rest. Not too shabby. Your body is actually giving you a bonus for exercising. It is saying to you, "Well, if you are smart enough to exercise, then you deserve a bonus for your good work." Your body is a wonderful machine and it gives you a reward for using, and not abusing it. Your body is actually saying to you, "Lets work together toward good health, physical fitness, and weight loss, and if you exercise and keep our metabolism revved up, then I will keep the motor going when you stop to rest." I would say that is a unique combination that is impossible to beat.

30 MINUTES OF WALKING POWERS THE DIETWALK

Thirty minutes walking briskly (approximately 3.5 mph) every day except Sunday is all you need to do for the exercise component of the DIETWALK Plan. Either 30 minutes outdoors (walking) or 30 minutes indoors (stationary bike or treadmill) will provide you with maximum cardiovascular fitness, good health, and boundless energy. Remember, this 30-minute walk is a basic part of your weight loss program. Your 30-minute walk, 6 days per week, is what burns the extra calories needed to lose additional weight and to decrease your appetite. The walking plan also provides the fuel that powers your energy level throughout your day. **When you combine 30 minutes of walking with the DietWalk Plan, you have the added power to burn additional calories.**

THE EXERCISE FALLACIES

Why are there so many exercise dropouts? And why don't many men and women even try to begin an exercise plan in the first place? Most people think that an exercise program is futile, since they'll never be able to look like the perfect bodies in the magazines or at the gym. You don't have to be put into a situation where you feel intimidated by an instructor in a gym or on a DVD.

Most people think physical fitness is actually harder than it is. And they feel that exercise programs are too complicated, when they hear terms like "oxygen consumption," "body fat composition," "body mass index," "lean muscle mass," etc. It all sounds too complicated and too boring for most men and women to begin exercising in any formalized program.

What most people don't realize is that you don't have to participate in a regimented exercise program to see results. You don't have to join a gym or health club and be intimidated by a twenty-year-old fitness instructor with boundless energy. And you don't have to exercise vigorously or do strenuous exercises in order to obtain maximum fitness and to develop a lean, trim body. As we've already discussed, exercise doesn't have to be strenuous to be beneficial. Also, exercise doesn't have to be painful in order to be gainful. Exercise can really be fun! It can be easy to follow and easy to continue. It doesn't have to be boring or a drudgery that has to be done. That's why the DietWalk Plan was devised—in order to make it easy for people to become fit and trim, and to make it easy for them to maintain their new level of fitness.

There are two main fallacies about exercising that you should be aware of. The first is the **"No Pain—No Gain"** myth, which is completely false. An exercise doesn't have to be painful to be beneficial. In fact, the reverse is actually true: moderate exercise is more beneficial than strenuous exercise.

The second fallacy is the **"Target Heart Rate Zone"** myth. No one has ever proved that you have to get your heart rate up to astronomical numbers to insure cardiovascular fitness. Here the reverse is also true: moderate exercise provides better cardiovascular fitness than strenuous exercise. Both of these so-called exercise precepts are what make women discontinue their exercise plans or never start them in the first place. Once you realize that both of these concepts are fallacies or myths and that it is not necessary to make exercise painful or stressful, you can begin to begin to relax and enjoy the **DIETWALK Plan.**

OTHER COMMON EXERCISE MYTHS ADDRESSED

If you're exercising strenuously, and you're breathing rapidly and shallowly during your exercise, then you're not delivering enough oxygen into the lungs, where it can be absorbed into the bloodstream. If, however, you walk at a moderately brisk pace, and take longer deeper breaths while exercising, you're able to deliver more oxygen deep into your lung tissues, and thus absorb more oxygen into your bloodstream.

Be careful when increasing your walking speed, and resist the temptation to stretch your stride too far. If you stretch your stride too far, then you will throw off your balance while walking, and put extra stress on your knees and shinbones.

There is no such thing as *spot reduction* while doing different exercises. For instance, you won't remove fat deposits in your buttocks on a stair climber or elliptical machine. Also, doing sit-ups won't remove excess fat around your waist. When you follow a healthy low fat, high fiber diet, combined with a well-rounded exercise program like walking or walking with light hand-held weights, fat will be burned gradually from fat deposits all over your body.

DIETWALK WALKING TIPS

1. Our bodies are one of the few machines that break down when not in use. A physically active person is one who is both physically and mentally alert. A walking program can actually slow down the aging process and add years to our lives. Walking has been proven to be a significant factor in the prevention of heart and vascular disease. It strengthens the heart muscle, improves the lung's efficiency, and lowers the blood pressure by keeping the blood vessels flexible. Walking will add years to your life, and life to your years!

2. In order to walk comfortably and efficiently without tiring, you should balance your body weight over the feet or just slightly ahead of them. Keep your body relaxed, and your knees bent slightly, utilizing a steady, even pace, and a brisk walking stride. To obtain the most benefit out of your walking program you should try to walk with the DietWalk® heel-and-toe method, pointing your feet straight ahead. By utilizing this method, your leg muscles are used more efficiently, and this results in an overall increased blood supply to the peripheral circulation (in particular the legs and feet) and to the general circulation (all of the body's cells, tissues and organs).

3. The leading leg is brought forward in front of the body, thus enabling the heel of the lead foot to touch the ground just before the ball of the foot and the toes. Your weight is then shifted forward so that when your heel is raised, your toes will push off for the next step. Your arms and shoulders should be

relaxed, and they will swing automatically with each stride you take. Before long, you will develop a natural rhythm, pace, and stride as you walk. The DietWalk® walking method uses the calf muscles to pump the blood up the leg veins back to the heart and lungs, and then out through the arteries to all your body's cells, tissues, and organs. This walking method keeps your body lean and your arteries clean.

4. When you walk, don't slouch. Walk tall! The way to walk is with your head up, shoulders back, stomach in, and your chest out. Learning to walk tall comes with practice, but after a while, this stance will become a natural part of your walking style. Your stride is the single most important aspect of your walk.

5. There is no correct stride length. Stretch as much as you can without straining when you are walking. Thrust your legs forward briskly, swing your arms vigorously and feel your energy surge forth as you walk with an even, effortless stride.

6. Keep your pace steady, never push and don't try to accelerate your speed when walking. If you do get tired after a short period of time, stop and rest and then restart again at a steady and even pace. Don't rush; just walk at a comfortable pace. Your rhythm of walking is a condition that will come naturally as you continue your walking program. Keep your body relaxed and your stride steady and even, and your rhythm will develop naturally. Uneven walking surfaces that you encounter will control your rhythm, especially going down or uphill. Don't fight it, just walk naturally and you'll be doing the DietWalk.

7. The DietWalk walking method is the ideal weight control and fitness program. Studies in human physiology have proven that walking acts as a weight reduction plan without actually dieting and a fitness program without strenuous exercises. Too often today we allow a sedentary lifestyle to dominate our daily living. We sit at our desks all day and in front of the TV set in the evenings. We drive to our destination, no matter how close or how far, instead of doing what's easy, natural and healthful—walking. Most of us would rather spend 20 minutes in our cars

waiting at the drive-in window of a bank, rather than getting out and walking the length of the parking lot. Even at work, we opt for the elevator even if it's only for a few floors. At the supermarket or shopping mall most of us would rather drive around the parking lot several times, so that we can get a parking spot closer to the store. These are all good opportunities to do the DietWalk. Use your feet, not your wheels, and you'll look great and feel full of pep when you walk.

8. Remember, it's the amount of *time* (30 minutes) that you walk every day that is more important than the distance or even the speed of walking. Even though the average walking speed for most people is approximately 3 miles per hour, it doesn't really make any difference whether you are walking 2½, 3, or 3½ per hour. You are still burning calories, losing weight, and developing physical fitness. In other words, it doesn't matter how far you walk or how fast you walk, as long as you walk regularly. You'll be walking for 30 minutes, 6 days each week to keep your fitness and energy level at its peak. When you begin walking, your respiration and heart rate will automatically become faster; however, if you feel short-of-breath or tired, then you're probably walking too fast. Remember to stop whenever you are tired or fatigued and then resume walking after resting. Concentrate on walking naturally, putting energy into each step. Soon you will begin to feel relaxed and comfortable as your stride becomes smooth and effortless. Walk with an even, steady gait and your own rhythm of walking will automatically develop into an unconscious synchronous movement.

9. When you first start your walking program, pick a level terrain, since hills place too much strain and stress on your legs, hips, and back muscles. Concentrate on maintaining erect posture while walking. Walk with your shoulders relaxed and your arms carried in a relatively low position with natural motion at the elbow. Don't hold your arms too high when you walk, otherwise you will develop muscle spasms and pain in your neck, back, and shoulder muscles.

BOOST YOUR ENERGY LEVEL

Once you've started walking for 30 minutes, six days per week, you will begin to notice the many changes brought about by your improved aerobic fitness and maximum oxygen capacity (the uptake and distribution of oxygen through your body). You will have lots of pep and energy, a trim figure, improved breathing capacity and muscle tone, improved exercise tolerance, a better night's sleep, a feeling of peace and relaxation, and a lessening of tension. Once you have completed this 21-day conditioning program, you will have taken the first steps towards improved cardiovascular fitness, good health, and a long, happy life. Then all you need to do is to *walk 30 minutes every day except Sunday (or any free day of the week) to reap all of the fitness and calorie burning benefits of the DietWalk Plan.*

The great part about walking as an exercise is that you aren't limited to a particular time or location. Walking doesn't require special clothes or equipment. You can walk before or after work, or if you drive to work, you can park your car a block or two from the office, and walk the rest of the way. If you take the bus or train, get off a stop before your station and walk. An enclosed mall could be the perfect place for your walk in bad weather. Remember to take 30 minutes from your lunch break and walk. Just think of how good that fresh air will feel and smell. Each city or town usually has a guidebook containing historical sites, restaurants, shops of interest, cultural centers, and interesting walking paths or tours. If you live near a park, the country or the seashore, a walking trip will be a refreshing change. Take the time to walk everywhere. Each new area has its own natural beauty.

The wonderful world of walking is literally at your feet. Just take that next step for vigor, vim, and pep.

INDOOR DIETWALK® PLAN

It's not necessary to wait until the "weather is better" to go out and walk. There's no excuse for not exercising at home on any day when the weather is inclement. Also, take precautions against exercising when it's very hot or humid outdoors. Heat exhaustion and occasionally heat stroke are complications frequently found in those fanatical runners that you see running on hot, humid days. Remember, it's not necessary to walk outdoors if the weather is extremely cold, windy, wet, hot, or humid. Here are various indoor exercise alternatives to help you stay on your DietWalk Plan.

STATIONARY DIETWALK

This is a combination of walking and running in place. Walk in place for 5 minutes, lifting your foot approximately 4 inches off the floor and taking approximately 60 steps a minute (count only when right foot hits floor). Alternate this with 5 minutes of running in place, lifting your foot approximately 8 inches off the floor and taking approximately 90 steps a minute (again only count when the right foot hits the floor). Use a padded exercise mat or a thick rug. Wear a padded sneaker or walking shoe. Bare feet will cause foot and leg injuries. Repeat this walk-run cycle twice daily, for a total of 35 minutes. If you tire easily, stop and rest.

DIETWALK DANCE

Turn on the music and dance to your favorite music, whether it's pop, jazz, classical, R&B, or any music with a moderately fast beat. Make up your own moves and dance to the beat of the music.

MUSIC BURNS STRESS AND CALORIES

Music can release stress and tension and alleviate anxiety by focusing your thoughts on the music rather than on your problem. Portable CD players or Ipods can actually push people to exercise harder. Walking to music helps you to burn more calories and lose more weight while relieving stress and tension.

You can create your own mix of songs to include a warm-up phase, some fast-paced tunes and mellow music for your cool-down phase.

Music in the range of 115 to 120 beats per minute is ideal for walking. Computers are able to calculate a song's beat per minute, letting people create music that is suitable for their own individual workout. For instance, if you like to walk faster than three miles per hour, then choose music with more than 120 beats per minute. If you do not want to bother to calculate a song's beat per minute, then let your body naturally adjust to the beat of the individual song you are listening to.

You can also work out at home to music while on your stationary bike or treadmill. The faster the music, the faster your workout and the more calories you will burn. If you are not into indoor exercise machines, then try dancing to the music at home. Dancing is a whole-body exercise that can be as gentle or as vigorous as you like. Any type of dance step will do. It is your preference whether it is tap, jazz, folk, modern or aerobic dance. You can usually find a video that helps you dance to your favorite type of dance step.

In a study at Farley Dickinson University it was shown that women who exercise to music, in addition to lowering their calorie intake, lost twice the amount of fat and pounds compared to a group of women who did not listen to music when they exercised. It was thought that the music exercising women were more motivated and pushed themselves harder during their exercise program than those women who did not listen to music while exercising.

STATIONARY BIKE DIETWALK

One of the easiest ways to continue your indoor DietWalk program is by using a stationary exercise bicycle. This is the only one-time investment you'll ever need to make as you travel the road toward fitness and good health. No other type of exercise equipment is necessary for your DietWalk program.

The most important features to look for in a stationary bicycle are a comfortable seat with good support, adjustable handlebars, a chain guard, a quiet pedal and chain, and a solid front wheel. Most come with speedometers to tell the rate that you are pedaling and odometers to tell the mileage that you pedal. An inexpensive stationary bike works just as well as an expensive one. Stationary bikes with moving handlebars are worthless. They claim to exercise the upper half of your body. In reality, they move your arms and back muscles passively, which can result in pulled muscles and strained ligaments.

The stationary bike is the safest and most efficient type of indoor exercise equipment that can be used in place of your outdoor walking program. You can listen to music, watch TV, talk on the telephone, or even read (a bookstand attachment can easily be clamped onto the handle bars) while riding your stationary bike. If the bike comes with a tension dial, leave it on zero or minimal tension. Remember, it is not necessary to strain yourself to develop aerobic fitness. Exercises like walking and the stationary bike can be fun, without being painful or stressful. You may alternate days of outdoor walking and indoor cycling depending on your individual schedule.

You should pedal at a comfortable rate of between 10-15 miles/ hour. To complete your daily exercise requirements, pedal for 30 minutes every day (divide into two sessions to avoid fatigue). Always wear a walking shoe or sneaker (never pedal barefoot). A chain guard prevents clothing from getting caught in the bike chain; otherwise roll up your sweats.

RECUMBENT STATIONARY BIKES

Some people feel that their body alignment is more comfortable and natural on a recumbent stationary bike. They also tend to say that the bike seats are more comfortable and ergonomically shaped than seats for upright bikes. Some studies have also shown that the recumbent stationary bike puts less stress on the upper and lower back muscles while pedaling. Recumbent bikes also help to build up the quadriceps muscles more than stationary upright bikes because of the leg positioning, and are therefore good for individuals with knee problems. It's an individual choice as to which type of bike feels most comfortable for you. Both bikes provide the same level of aerobic fitness and calorie burning.

TREADMILLS

The treadmill is an effective way to burn calories and build cardiovascular fitness. Manual treadmills are hard on the feet, since you have to push down to make them move and the walking motion is unnatural. Look for motorized treadmills with a deck area (the walking space) with enough length and width to accommodate any stride. The deck area should be at least 18 inches wide by 55 inches long. A cushioned deck is better for your ankles and knees and a thick tread belt is best. You can compare the thickness by the feel when you try out the treadmill or by asking the salesman for the thickness measurement.

Look for motorized treadmills with a high continuous duty rating of at least 1.5 horsepower as opposed to a motor with a maximum output. Continuous duty motors give you constant maximum power, whereas maximum output motors surge to accommodate short spurts, but you won't be able to walk smoothly for an extended period of time. You can also choose a treadmill with a power incline; however, too much of an incline is bad for the knees and ankles and can put a strain on your back. Also, make sure that the machine has an automatic stop button, since, if you stumble or feel dizzy, you can push the button and halt the machine instantly. Exercise for 35 minutes a day either at one time, or divided into two sessions. Some people find that the treadmill is too hard on their knees, because of the constant pounding and impact that the legs endure. An elliptical machine may be a better choice for these individuals.

WALKING WHILE WORKING EXERCISE

Many women and men spend much of the day in front of their computers. It's often difficult to find time during the day to go to a gym, and many people are too tired after a long day at the office to exercise, even at home. There is a unique alternative that will allow you to walk while you are working. It has been shown that you can set up a *slow-moving treadmill* in front of your workstation. Your workstation should be mounted above your treadmill by creating a shelf for your laptop. This type of indoor exercise may be too complicated for most people; however, many business people who don't have the time to exercise during the day have utilized this combo of work and exercise.

You have to go slow on the treadmill at first (approximately 0.5 miles per hour) so that you can type or read without bopping up and down. Set your laptop on the shelf so that your eyes are level with the middle of the screen and your forearms are parallel to the floor. This procedure may take a lot of practice before you can get used to it; however, once mastered, you can burn a lot of calories during the day without sitting at your desk workstation.

To get started, start the process while watching TV first, and then graduate to surfing the Internet, so that you can feel comfortable with your computer. Then gradually start to type, send, and receive emails. Follow that process with actually doing your regular work on your computer while walking on the treadmill. For additional tips on this unique form of workout, check out websites such as: www.walking-whileworking.com. You don't need an expensive treadmill for this activity, since you won't be using it for running.

This type of walking while working exercise can also be accomplished using an *upright stationary bike,* where you hook up your laptop computer to the front of the bike on a stand. Many stationary bikes come with built in stands for books, which can be widened to accommodate a computer. Also, remember an additional benefit of walking or riding while working. Work related telephone calls can easily be accomplished while you're exercising. In fact, the added endorphins produced while exercising will give you the added benefit of clear and insightful thinking during your business calls. Many great ideas and plans have been generated by the person who walks or rides while working.

ELLIPTICAL FITNESS MACHINES

This type of machine combines the movement of a treadmill and a stair climber. Your feet loop forward to simulate walking, but the footpads rise and fall with your feet. The elliptical motion provides a no-impact type of exercise, which is great if you have arthritis or knee or back problems that make walking difficult. For maximum exercise, an elliptical machine with dual cross-trainer arms, which move back and forth as you stride, rather than the stationary arms, provides maximum exercise and burns more calories and uses more muscle groups. Most of these machines come with an adjustable ramp incline and resistance settings. However, the normal setting is usually more than adequate for cardiovascular fitness. Also, be careful of small space-saving elliptical machines, since they may not comfortably accommodate a tall person's stride, or may not afford full range of motion. Try out different machines to see which one is most comfortable. The elliptical machine can be a very good alternative to outdoor walking. It's best to divide this exercise into two sessions, totaling 30 minutes.

Swimming

Thirty minutes of swimming provides the same aerobic conditioning and cardiovascular fitness benefits as walking and other indoor Fit-Step exercises. Swimming has the added benefit of being easy on the joints, especially if you have any form of arthritis or back problems. Swimming puts very little stress on the joints because of the decreased gravity factor provided by the buoyancy of the water. If you have access to an indoor or outdoor swimming pool, then 35 minutes of swimming will fit the bill perfectly for the DietWalk plan. Water aerobics are excellent non-weight-bearing exercises for fitness, weight-loss, body shaping, and for helping to prevent osteoporosis.

Skipping Dietwalk

If you're coordinated enough to use a jump rope, skipping can be a fun indoor exercise. Skip over the rope alternating one foot at a time for 5 minutes and then skip using both feet together for 10 minutes. Use a mat or padded rug with a padded low sneaker or walking shoe. Do this exercise two or three times daily for a total of 30 minutes. If you feel you are not coordinated enough for rope skipping, then skip it!

Mall Walking

For those of you who don't like to exercise at home when the weather's bad, an indoor mall can be just the place to take your 30-minute walk. Many malls open early before the stores open to accommodate "mall walkers." If you have access to one of these enclosed malls and don't like to stay at home exercising, then by all means, get out there and do the Fit-Step®. Remember to put vigor, vim, and pep into your mall walk step. Keep your eyes straight ahead so that you won't be window shopping walking. If you tire easily, then divide your walk into two sessions, totaling 35 minutes.

TRAVEL FIT WITH DIETWALK

Whether you're taking a vacation or a business trip, you can still keep trim and fit with your walking program. Most major airlines, cruise ships and trains offer special diet menus. If you have to splurge on one meal a day, don't worry. You'll walk it off in no time at all. Cruise ships and trains are ideal for short walks. Walk around the airport concourse while waiting for flights or during layovers. Most major hotels can give you a map of the area for a walking tour. Get up early before your meeting and take a brisk 30-minute walk. Use the stairs whenever possible and walk around the hotel as much as possible if the weather is bad.

Many hotels have small gyms where you can swim or use a stationary bike; take advantage of them if the weather's bad instead of watching TV. Many business trips are associated with a lot of stress and walking can ease away the tension, leaving you more relaxed and more efficient. Speakers always do better after they've had a walk— more brain oxygen and relaxing chemicals (endorphins) and less carbon dioxide result in a sharp, clear, concise speech with no stage jitters. You can keep fit and have lots of pep when you do the DietWalk. Don't let a little trip, trip you up. Most people feel exhausted after a vacation or a business trip because they sit around all day and stuff their faces with food and drink. Make it a habit to walk at least 30 minutes every day that you're away. You'll return from your travels fit, full of vigor, vim and pep.

WALKING FOR FITNESS AND FUN

1. Be sure to get a complete physical exam from your physician before starting any exercise program.

2. Never exercise if you are injured or ill. Your body needs time to heal and recuperate from whatever ails you. Remember, you can't exercise through an injury or an illness. Many so-called fitness-nuts have tried this with disastrous results. For example, a strained muscle has been aggravated into a fractured bone or a simple cold has turned into pneumonia. Listen to your body.

3. Keep a record of your walking program. For example, how long did you walk today, and approximately how far did you walk? Record the time and location of your walk and your impressions of the area in which you walked. Maybe it's an area you'd like to stay away from or one you'd like to explore again.

4. Record your weight only once every week to see if you are losing the amount of weight you'd like to lose, or if you are just walking to maintain your present weight. Remember walkers who want to maintain their present weight usually can have a bonus snack every day without gaining an ounce.

5. Don't expect results too soon. Whether it's fitness or weight-control that you're looking for, remember, "Rome wasn't built in a day and neither were you." Give your body time to adapt to your regular walking program.

6. Vary your walking program. Vary your walking times (morning, afternoon or evening) depending on your schedule.

7. Make your walking program convenient and flexible. The more adaptable you are to when and where you walk, the more likely you are to do it on a regular basis.

8. Either walk alone or with a friend or relative. Walking can be a social activity as well as an exercise. Spending time with someone you like or love can certainly add to the enjoyment of your walking program. Walking is one of the only exercises that lets you talk as you walk. If you are unable to talk because of shortness of breath, then you're probably walking too fast.

9. Change your walking route every week or two. If near home or work, walk in a different direction, and observe, feel and smell new sights, sounds, and odors on your new route. The road less traveled may be the most fun.

10. Take a walk-break instead of a coffee-break. Walking actually clears the mind and puts vitality and energy back into your body's walking machine. Coffee and a donut add caffeine and sugar to your body's sitting machine. Both the caffeine

and sugar cause your insulin production to be increased, and following an initial rise in blood sugar, there is a sharp drop in your blood sugar from this excess insulin. So instead of coming back to work invigorated as you do from a walk break, you come back fatigued, light-headed and dizzy from a coffee and donut-break.

11. Wear a pedometer, which keeps track of the miles that you walk. Particularly good computerized pedometers will measure steps taken, distance traveled, calories burned, pace, heart rate, and timed events.

12. Buy a good walking shoe that fits properly and has good support and adequate cushioning for comfortable walking.

13. Don't be afraid to take a break for a few days or even a week. Any exercise program, even one as easy and fun-filled as walking, can eventually become a little tiring. A few days' break from your schedule will give you a short breather so that you can return to your walking program with renewed interest and enthusiasm. Remember, you won't gain all of your weight back or get out of shape if you take an occasional break from your walking program.

14. Even though walking is the safest and most hazard-free exercise known to women, it is still essential that you have a complete physical examination by your family physician before starting your walking program. It is essential that you follow your own individual doctor's recommendations before beginning any exercise program, including a walking program, especially if you have a history of any medical condition.

TAKE A HAPPY WALK

Americans are walking again like never before. According to the President's Council on Physical Fitness report, walking is the single most popular adult exercise in America. With over 52 million adherents, the numbers are steadily increasing as men and women of all ages are walking for health, fitness, and fun. Walking is an exercise whose time has finally come. Why not? It's easy, safe, fun, and it makes you feel and look great.

Walking is something that two people, no matter how different their physical conditions, can do together. It is a companionable exercise in which you enjoy each other's company and at the same time get all the benefits of exercising. Walking is a great escape. You can get away from the phone, from the office, or from home for a little while, and take that needed time to relax. You can walk to think out a problem or walk to forget one. Walking acts as a tranquilizer to help us relax and it can work as a stimulant to give us energy. The late famous cardiologist Dr. Paul Dudley White said, "*A vigorous 3-mile walk will do more for an unhappy but otherwise healthy adult than all the medicine and psychology in the world.*" Don't make the common mistake of thinking that walking is too easy to be a good exercise. On the contrary, walking is not only the safest, but it's the best exercise in the world. If you're overweight, then walking is your best choice since you won't be putting excessive stress on the ligaments, muscles, and joints.

How you walk also tells whether you're happy, sad, angry, ambitious, or just plain lazy. Walkers with a long stride, a greater arm swing, and a bounce to their step are happy, ambitious, and self-assured, whereas walkers with a short stride, foot shuffle or drag, and a short arm swing are often depressed, unhappy, and angry. Recent studies in women indicate that arm swing is the most indicative factor of their mood. The greater the arm swing, the happier, more vigorous, and less depressed a person is. A short arm swing indicated that a person was angry, frustrated, and unhappy. Stretch out your stride, swing your arms, and put a bounce in your step whenever and wherever you walk. That's your road to good health, a successful career, and a long, happy life. Believe it! It works!

I'M GIVING UP! EXERCISE IS BORING

How many times have you heard someone (or even perhaps yourself) say, **"I'm giving up, exercise is boring!"** Over 65% of women who start an exercise program abandon it after 4-6 weeks. Surprising, isn't it? Not really! Initial enthusiasm is often quickly replaced by boredom. Most of the exercise equipment and athletic clothes quickly find their way into the recesses of the closet.

Walking, fortunately, is one of the only exercises that the majority of people stay with. The percentage of women who give up walking as a regular form of exercise is less than 25% of those who start on a walking program. Perhaps it's because walking doesn't require special equipment or clothing. Or perhaps it's because there are no clubs to join or dues to pay. Or perhaps it's just that most walkers are usually rugged individualists and are more determined than most to keep in good shape.

I think the real reason that walkers stay with their walking program is simply that walking is fun! And isn't that what an exercise should be? True, we all want physical fitness, good health, weight control, and longevity. But we also want an escape from the stress of everyday living, and that's simply having fun. Walking provides a stress-free, fun-filled activity that we can do anyplace, anywhere, anytime whatsoever.

STAY MOTIVATED

Most women who are overweight or not physically fit are usually too embarrassed to join a gym. Joining a gym should be the last thing on your mind. All you have to do is take a brisk walk for 30 minutes six days per week, and you're on your way to losing weight and becoming physically fit. If you can't fit 30 minutes at one time into your daily schedule, then try to divide it into 2 or 3 sessions a day. Your weight-loss and fitness benefits will be exactly the same as one 30-minute daily walk.

Staying motivated is the key to any successful weight-loss and fitness program. Walking with a companion is one way to stay motivated. Also, varying the route and location of your walk every couple of days will give you a fresh perspective on your daily walking exercise. You'll be exposed to new sights, sounds and smells, such as a park with pretty, fragrant flowers and beautiful trees. Also, you'll see different sections of the city or suburbs that you live or work in with a variety of new faces and places. It's easy to stay motivated with the

DietWalk Plan, since you will find new and exciting places to walk every day no matter what city or town that you live in.

Another sure-fire way to stay motivated when you walk is to vary the speed or intensity of walking during your walking exercise workout. For instance, speed up your walking pace for 30-60 seconds every 5 to 10 minutes during your 30-minute walk. You'll feel the extra energy pour into your body as you take in additional oxygen with your increased speed of walking. You'll also burn more calories as you speed up your walk, thus increasing your rate of weight-loss and physical fitness. Also, if you walk an extra 5 or 10 minutes a day, you will vary your daily exercise routine as you burn more calories for additional weight-loss and fitness.

You'll be able to stay motivated when you add the Strength-Training Exercises, where you'll be walking for 30 minutes with light-weight, hand-held weights 3 times per week.

Chapter 8 describes this in more detail.

POWER WEIGHT LOSS WALKING STEPS

Walking on **softer surfaces** like sand, dirt, or grass could help you burn an extra 100 calories in 30 minutes. This type of activity should be limited to one or two days per week.

Walk up hills as part as of your walking program on two or three days per week. This can help you burn an additional 150 calories in 30 minutes.

Walking on cobblestones or **uneven surfaces** uses different muscles than walking on a flat surface and burns more calories as you walk. It is important to be careful to walk carefully on these uneven surfaces to prevent ankle and/or foot strains or sprains. Also, be careful of unfortunate trips and falls.

Intermittent speed walking—Walk as fast as you can for two minutes and then slow down to your normal three miles per hour pace. Increase speed again after five minutes of your normal pace for another two minutes. Do this three or four times during your 30-minute walk, depending on your fatigue level. If you become fatigued or short of breath, then just do your speed walking at one-minute intervals. If fatigue, shortness of breath, chest pain, or any other symptoms occur, discontinue speed walking and see your doctor immediately.

Walk up and down **stairs** ten minutes every day in addition to your 30-minute walking program. This will burn an additional 100 calories per day.

Increase your **speed of walking** from 3 to 4 miles per hour for 10 minutes, and then resume walking at three miles per hour. You can use a pedometer to calculate distance and speed of walking.

To **burn even more calories**, increase your speed from three miles per hour to 4 to 4.5 miles for ten minutes, and then resume your walk at three miles per hour.

Stretch your stride so that your foot lands first on your heel and then on your sole all the way through your stride to end up on your toes. This stretching of your stride tones and firms leg muscles and burns additional calories.

Concentrate on **holding your tummy in** while you walk for several minutes, and then release your abdominal muscles. This burns additional calories and helps to melt belly fat.

Increase your walking time 30 minutes daily to anywhere from 45-60 minutes every day. This could burn significantly more calories each day.

WHAT'S THE BEST TIME TO DO YOUR WALKING WORKOUT?

You can do your walking aerobic workout exercise any time of the day that's convenient for you. It's your schedule, so make it any time that you'd like. You can also change the times that you exercise each day depending on your own individual work schedule or home activities. Here are the pros and cons of exercising at various times of the day according to the so-called fitness experts. Take it with a grain of salt and individualize your own schedule to your own liking.

Morning—The main obstacle in the morning is getting out of bed. Once you're up, depending on if you're an early riser or not, you may want to leave yourself enough time so that you won't be rushed, especially if you have to go to work or have home responsibilities. Since there are usually few disruptions in the A.M., women and men who walk in the morning are more likely to stick with their exercise plans over a long period of time. Plus, the sense of accomplishment; having completed your exercise early in the day gives you a psychological rush for the first part of the day.

Afternoon—Many people feel an energy lag between two and three P.M. in the afternoon, which is related to the body's natural circadian rhythm. It may also be partly due to having just eaten lunch. Some exercise physiologists say that walking mid-day can smooth out that energy lag by increasing the levels of certain hormones that will perk you up for several hours. Remember, however, that it is not a good idea to exercise immediately after lunch or to skip lunch altogether. Walking for 25 minutes and then eating a light lunch will boost your energy level for the rest of the day.

Evening—Due to fluctuations in biological rhythms, it is in the late afternoon or early evening when your breathing is easier because your lungs' airways open wider, your muscle strength increases due to a slightly higher body temperature, and your joints and muscles are at their most flexible. This may also be a good time to walk according to some exercise physiologists. However, if you've had an extremely difficult day, and if you're dead tired, then revving yourself up for exercise may seem more like a chore than fun. Also, never exercise near bedtime, since the increased energy levels that follow the exercise may make it difficult to fall asleep. Determine the best time to do the DietWalk workout according to your own biological clock and how you feel, and also according to your own time schedule. It's your body, so listen to it, and it will respond to you with boundless energy and pep when you do the DietWalk.

CHAPTER SIX RAPID READ

- *30 minutes of aerobic walking 6 days per week;* The aerobic walking program for 30 minutes causes your body's metabolism to burn calories during and also after you're walking.

- Moderate exercise is more beneficial and provides better cardiovascular fitness than strenuous exercise.

- The amount of *time* (30 minutes) that you walk every day is more important than the distance or even the speed of walking.

- Indoor exercise alternatives to help you stay on your DietWalk Plan include walking in place, dancing, using a stationary bike, treadmill, or elliptical trainer, swimming, skipping rope, or walking in malls.

- Staying motivated is the key to any successful weight-loss and fitness program. Walking with a companion is one way to stay motivated; vary the route and location of your walk; vary the speed or intensity of walking; add the Strength-Training Exercises

You can burn additional calories by

- Walking on **softer surfaces** (an extra 100 calories/30 minutes).

- **Walk up hills** (an additional 150 calories/30 minutes).

- Walk up and down **stairs** ten minutes every day in addition to your 30-minute walking program (an additional 100 calories/day).

- Increase your **speed of walking**.

- Concentrate on **holding your tummy in** while you walk for several minutes, and then release your abdominal muscles.

- Increase your walking time 30 minutes

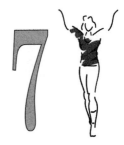

Power Weight Loss

THE FAT FORMULA

The latest report from the National Institute of Health again confirmed that obesity is a major health risk. The evidence is strong that obesity not only shortens life, but actually affects the quality of life also. Almost 20 percent of Americans are overweight. How can you tell if you're one of them? It's simple—just follow the **fat formula** for your normal weight:

> **Females**—100 lbs. for the first 5 feet in height, plus 5 lbs. for each additional inch. Example: 5'2" = 110 lbs.

> **Males**—106 lbs. for the first 5 feet in height, plus 6 lbs. for each additional inch. Example: 5' 9" = 160 lbs.

BMI

Body mass index (BMI) is a measurement of your weight related to your height. It is another way to assess body fat. The BMI is a complicated mathematical formula based on your weight in pounds and your height in inches. It's much easier to consult BMI tables on the Internet or in health magazines than to try to figure out this mathematical formula yourself. Generally, the BMI also rates your risk of heart disease depending on your body mass index. The following is a general chart **(Table I),** which indicates if you're overweight and your potential risk of heart disease.

TABLE I: Heart Disease Risk

BMI	WEIGHT	HEART DISEASE RISK
18.5-24.9	Normal	None
25.0-29.9	Overweight	Increased
30.0-34.0	Minimal Obesity	High
35.0-39.9	Moderate Obesity	Very High
40.0 or greater	Extremely Obese	Extremely High

If you flunk the fat formula or the BMI, then you really need to start to walking off weight using the **QUICK WEIGHT-LOSS WALKING PLANS.** The increased medical risks for being overweight are: hypertension, heart attacks, strokes, diabetes, arthritis, cancer of all types, and increased surgical risks if you happen to need an operation. These risks seem to be even worse if most of your weight is carried in the upper body (chest, hips, and abdomen) rather than in the buttocks and legs.

QUICK WEIGHT-LOSS WALKING

The Fit-Step: 30-Minute Plan was based on walking at a brisk pace (3.5 mph) for 30 minutes six days per week, combined with the **Diet-Step Plan: 30/30 Plan.** This weight-loss program is based upon the number of calories burned by the combination of dieting and walking. Walking at 3.5 miles per hour is a speed that can be maintained for a long duration without causing stress, strain, or fatigue. We are not talking about window-shopping walking, which is much too slow (1 to 2 miles/hr.) and is not at all useful in burning calories. Nor are we suggesting fast walking (4-5 miles/hr.), which is too fast to be continued for long periods of time without tiring. And we certainly are not recommending race walking (5 to 6 miles/hr.), which is worthless as a permanent weight reduction plan, and has all of the same hazards and dangers that jogging has.

By following **The Quick Weight-Loss Walking Plans,** you will lose additional weight by walking off more pounds. This faster weight loss occurs because you will be walking more than just the 30 minutes, 6 days/week. The following Quick Weight-Loss Plans have been designed for faster weight-loss than the weight that you lose on the Diet-Step & Fit-Step Combination Plan. You can walk anywhere, anytime, anyplace, as long as you make the time.

All this additional weight loss occurs without your changing one thing in your **Diet- Step/Fit-Step combination diet and exercise plan**, except the time you walk each day. You will no longer just be walking for just 40 minutes, 6 days per week.

By following any one of these three Quick Weight-Loss Walking Plans, you will be able to lose more weight than you can lose on the Diet-Step/Fit-Step combination plan alone.

WANT TO LOSE WEIGHT FASTER?

Most women are more likely to perceive themselves as fat, whereas in reality, men are more likely to be overweight. In a recent Harris poll of over 1,200 women and men nationwide, the findings were as follows:

- Over 50% of women considered themselves overweight, compared to 38% of men.

- 65% of the men were actually overweight, compared with 62% of the woman.

- Almost 40% of those people surveyed stated that they were on a diet.

- 60% of those surveyed were overweight, which was exactly the same percentage as last year's survey.

- More than 50% of those surveyed felt they weren't getting enough exercise.

It doesn't appear that we're getting any thinner despite all of the diet books, health clubs, fitness centers, and diet promoters! So, what's the answer? Walking, of course! Walkers, by and large, are the least overweight segment of any population group. This fact has been verified in numerous medical studies.

"I DON'T REALLY EAT THAT MUCH!"

The question I get asked most often from patients about being overweight is, "How come I keep gaining weight? I don't really eat that much." Well, the truth of the matter is that we get heavier as we get older because our physical activity tends to decrease even though our food intake stays the same. The only way to beat the battle of the bulge is to burn those unwanted pounds away. Walking **burns calories**. The following table will give you an idea as to the energy expended in walking (**TABLE II**).

TABLE II: CALORIES BURNED BY WALKING

Walking Speed	Calories Burned/ Minute	Calories Burned/30 Minutes	Calories Burned/ Hour
Slow Speed (2 mph)	3-4	90-120	180-240
Moderate Speed (3 mph)	4-5	120-150	240-300
Brisk Speed (3.5 mph)	**5-6**	**150-180**	**300-360**
Fast Speed (4 mph)	6-7	180-210	360-420
Race Walking (5 mph)	7-8	210-240	420-480

A pound of body fat contains approximately 3,500 calories. When you eat 3,500 more calories than your body actually needs, it stores up that pound as body fat. If you reduce your intake by 3,500 calories, you will lose a pound. It doesn't make any difference how long it takes your body to store or burn these 3,500 calories. The result is always the same. You either gain or lose one pound of body fat, depending on how long it takes you to accumulate or burn up 3,500 calories.

You can then actually lose weight by just walking. When you walk at a speed of 3 mph for one hour every day, you will burn up **350 calories each day.** Therefore, if you walk for 30 minutes every day you will burn up 3,500 calories in 20 days. If you walk for 60 minutes a day you will burn up 3,500 calories in 10 days. Since there are 3,500 calories in each pound of fat, every time you burn up 3,500 calories by walking, you will lose a pound of body fat.

POWER WEIGHT-LOSS PLANS

POWER WEIGHT-LOSS PLAN # 1

- *Lose one additional pound every 20 days.*

On this **Power Weight-Loss plan** you will walk for **one hour every other day or ½ hour every day, 7 days per week.** Walking at a brisk pace of 3-3.5 mph, you will burn up approximately 350 calories every hour that you walk. Let's see how much weight you'll lose by this plan.

1. Walk ½ hour daily x 350 calories/hour = 175 calories burned per day.

2. Walk 3½ hours per week x 350 calories/hour = 1,225 calories burned per week.

3. Walk 10 hours every 20 days x 350 calories/hour = 3,500 calories burned or one pound lost every 20 days (or 175 cal. burned per day x 20 days = 3,500 calories).

On this walking-off-weight Power Weight-Loss plan you will lose one additional pound every 20 days, or 1½ extra pounds every month.

POWER WEIGHT-LOSS PLAN # 2

- *Lose one additional pound every 10 days.*

On this **Power Weight-Loss plan** you can lose one additional pound every 10 days just walking **one hour every day of the week.**

The only difference in this plan is that you are now walking an hour every day. You will still be burning up 350 calories every hour that you walk briskly (3 mph).

Since it takes 10 hours of walking at 3 mph to burn up 3,500 calories or one pound, if you walk for an hour every day, you will **lose one additional pound every 10 days.** By following this plan, you can actually **lose 3 extra pounds every month.**

POWER WEIGHT-LOSS PLAN # 3

* *Lose one additional pound every 7 days.*

For those of you who want to lose weight even faster, you can walk for **45 minutes twice daily.** By walking a total of 1½ hours every day of the week you will be able to speed up the walking-off-weight on this plan. When you walk 1½ hours every day, you will burn up 525 calories each day or 3,675 calories per week. You can see that you will lose a pound a week on this plan with a few extra (175 calories) to spare.

You may divide your 1½ hours of walking into three 30 minute sessions daily if that's more convenient for you. The weight-loss results will be the same. This plan will enable you to **lose one additional pound every week, or about 4 extra pounds a month.**

Again, all this additional weight loss occurs without your changing one thing in your **Diet-Step/Fit-Step combination diet and exercise plan**, except the time you walk each day. You will no longer just be walking for 30 minutes, 6 days per week.

By following any one of these three Power Weight-Loss plans, you will be able to lose more weight than you can lose on the Diet-Step/Fit-Step combination plan alone. This additional weight-loss occurs because you will be walking for longer periods of time every day. Remember, it's easy to lose more weight and look your best by just walking more every day.

POWER WEIGHT-LOSS SNACK PLAN

- *Snack on your favorite food—calorie free.*

Let's say your weight is just where you'd like it to be, but you don't want to gain another ounce. Or say your weight is nowhere near what you would like it to be, but you really can't afford to gain another pound without going into another size dress. Each of you would like to be able to cheat and at least stay the same weight. Well fear no more, the **Power Weight-Loss Snack Plan** is just for you.

How about a slice of cake, French fries, a cone of ice cream, a slice of pizza, a hamburger, or a glass of wine? With the **Power Weight-Loss Snack Plan** you have the perfect method that allows you to cheat without paying the price. Eat your favorite snack food, consult the following table (**TABLE III**) and walk the number of minutes listed in order to burn up the extra calories you've cheated on. The following table shows how many minutes of walking at a brisk pace (3 mph or 3½ mph) are necessary to burn up the caloric value of those foods listed.

If your favorite snack food is not listed on the following table, you can easily figure out the time you have to burn off your snack's calories. Look up the number of calories of your favorite snack food and divide by the number 6. This answer will give you the number of minutes it takes to walk off your snack. The number 6 comes from the fact that walking at a brisk pace (3 mph) burns approximately 6 calories per minute. Example: hamburger and roll = 438 calories. Divide 6 into 438 and you get 73. It will take you 73 minutes to walk of this snack.

TABLE III: QUICK WEIGHT-LOSS WALKING SNACK PLAN

(Time Required to Walk Off Snacks)	
American cheese (1 slice)	16 minutes
Apple (medium)	15 minutes
Apple juice (6 oz.)	17 minutes
Bagel (1)	23 minutes
Banana (medium)	16 minutes
Beer (12 oz.)	30 minutes

(Time Required to Walk Off Snacks)	
Bologna sandwich	50 minutes
Candy bar (1 oz.)	45 minutes
Cake (1 slice pound)	63 minutes
Chocolate bar/nuts (1 oz.)	28 minutes
Cheese crackers (6)	35 minutes
Cheese steak (½)	55 minutes
Chicken, fried (3 pieces)	50 minutes
Chocolate cookies (3)	25 minutes
Corn chips (small pack)	33 minutes
Doughnut (jelly)	40 minutes
Frankfurter & roll	50 minutes
French fries (3 oz.)	50 minutes
Hamburger (4 oz.) and roll	73 minutes
Ice cream cone	30 minutes
Ice cream sandwich	35 minutes
Ice cream sundae	75 minutes
Milk shake, chocolate (8 oz.)	42 minutes
Muffin, blueberry	25 minutes
Orange juice (6 oz.)	16 minutes
Peanut butter crackers (6)	50 minutes
Peanuts, in shell (2 oz.)	37 minutes
Pie, apple (1 slice)	46 minutes
Pizza (1 slice)	40 minutes
Potato chips (small pack)	33 minutes
Pretzels (hard—3 small)	30 minutes
Pretzels (soft—1 Superpretzel®)	30 minutes
Shrimp cocktail (6 small)	18 minutes
Soda-cola (12 oz.)	24 minutes
Tuna fish sandwich	41 minutes
Wine, Chablis (4 oz.)	14 minutes
Whiskey, rye (1 oz.)	17 minutes

EATING AND EXERCISE

As food enters your stomach, your heart pumps a significant quantity of blood into the stomach to aid in the digestive process. This does not pose a problem when you are at rest, but if you decide to exercise immediately after eating, then there is a conflict of interests. The stomach now has to compete with the exercising muscles for the blood it needs for digestion. If the exercise gets vigorous then digestion is arrested and you begin to feel bloated and develop abdominal cramps. Exercise should therefore begin after a meal has passed through the stomach and small intestines. This takes approximately 2 hours after ingesting a large meal and from 45-60 minutes after eating a smaller meal.

Foods high in saturated fat and unhealthy fatty protein are not efficient foods for energy production and tend to store excess fat in the body's fat cells. Foods that are high in refined sugar like cakes, candy, and pies can trigger an excess insulin response if they are eaten immediately before exercise. This means that the excess insulin produced as a result of the high sugar content of food, combined with the exertion of exercise, could drop the blood sugar rapidly. This could result in weakness, muscle cramps, and even fainting. On the other hand, foods that are higher in complex carbohydrates (whole-grain foods, vegetable, fruits) and healthy protein (lean meats, fish, white meat of chicken and turkey, non-fat dairy products, nuts, and seeds) tend to be absorbed slowly, thus avoiding the insulin spikes and the drops of blood sugar. These foods are efficient energy producers and burn calories steadily, so that no excess fat is stored in the body's fat cells.

On the other hand, fasting for long periods prior to exercise is in itself counterproductive. In order to replenish the energy stores (glycogen) in the liver and muscles, it is necessary to eat several hours before exercising. When you fast, you deplete these energy stores, and exercise then becomes difficult and tiring.

So, what does this all have to do with walking and eating? Very little, if anything. Most of these rules of digestion apply to strenuous and vigorous exercise with relation to mealtime. The most important fact to be learned from this discussion on digestive physiology is that it is essential that you don't walk immediately after eating, especially if you've consumed a relatively large meal (which you shouldn't be eating in the first place). This puts a strain on the cardiovascular system and can even deprive the heart of its own essential blood supply, particularly if you exercise vigorously immediately after eating (which you shouldn't be doing in the second place).

Walking 45-60 minutes after a small to moderate meal can actually aid in digestion, by nudging the foodstuffs gently along the digestive tract. This in no way competes for the blood in the digestive tract, since your walking muscles do not require nearly as much as strenuously exercising muscles require. In fact, the gentle art of walking allows oxygen to be evenly distributed to all of the body's internal organs, which in this particular case is the digestive tract.

Recent studies indicate a three-fold advantage for dieters who walk before and after meals. As we have previously seen, walking before eating slows down our appetite-control center in the brain and makes us less hungry. Secondly, walking at any time burns calories directly as we walk. And thirdly, new studies in exercise physiology have shown that walking anywhere from 45-60 minutes after eating a small to moderate-sized meal will actually burn 10-15% more calories than walking on an empty stomach. This is explained by a term called the **thermic dynamic action of food**. What this means is that the actual digestion of food products combined with the gentle action of walking results in a higher metabolic rate, thus burning more calories per hour. Also, because of this increase in your basal metabolic rate, your body actually continues to burn more calories after you walk than it does at rest alone.

EXERCISE INCREASES YOUR APPETITE: RIGHT?—WRONG!

Another myth regarding diet and exercise is that exercise stimulates the appetite. So, after you exercise you're hungry, and then you eat more, and you cancel out any calories you burned during exercise. Right? Wrong! Contrary to popular belief, walking actually decreases your appetite. It does this by several mechanisms that are described as follows:

1. **Walking burns fat rather than carbohydrates** and therefore does not drop the blood sugar precipitously. Strenuous exercises and calorie-reduction diets both drop the blood sugar rapidly, and it is this low blood sugar that stimulates your appetite and makes you hungry. Walking is a more moderate type of exercise and consequently burns fats slowly rather than carbohydrates quickly. This results in the blood sugar remaining constant. And when the blood sugar remains level, you do not feel hungry.

2. Walking also **increases the resting basal metabolic rate (BMR)**. This basal metabolic rate refers to the calories your body burns at rest in order to produce energy. When you go on a calorie restriction diet, your BMR slows. This is because your body assumes that the reduction in calories is the result of starvation and your body wants to burn fewer calories so you won't starve to death. The body has no way of knowing that you're on a diet. This is also one of the reasons that you don't continue to lose weight on a calorie reduction diet. The body prevents this excess weight loss by lowering its BMR, so you stop losing weight even though you are eating the same number of calories that you ate in the beginning of your diet.

3. Walking **redirects the blood supply** away from your stomach, toward the exercising muscles. With less blood supplied to the stomach, your appetite is reduced.

4. When you combine the **30 Gm Fat/ 30 Gm Fiber,** with 30 minutes of walking on the **30-Minute Dietwalk Plan**, then the walking component powers up your basal metabolic rate and causes you to burn more calories than if you were just following the diet alone. So in effect, walking prevents the BMR from decreasing and burning fewer calories, as when you only diet. The result: less hunger and more calories burned when you walk every day.

10,000 STEPS

In a recent study, researchers have discovered that walking approximately 10,000 steps a day is a threshold for physical fitness and weight loss. The women studied in this group wore pedometers every day to measure the number of steps they took. After a six-week period, the women who averaged 10,000 steps or more daily were found to have 35% less body fat and had lost 3-4 inches in their waist and hip measurements, compared to those women who took fewer than 6,000 steps per day. There are several other similar studies that have shown that both men and women who walked 10,000 steps or more daily not only lost weight, but also had significantly lower blood pressures

Six thousand steps means that you've walked approximately three miles. This appears to be the average number of steps that most active adults walk in a day, provided that they're not desk-bound for 8 hours daily. In order to add another 4,000 steps per day to this 6,000-step average, it would be necessary to walk for an additional 30 minutes a day. So here again we have more concrete proof that walking 30 minutes a day in addition to your regular activity is a great way to lose weight, get firm and fit, and boost energy. All you need to do is start and continue a regular 30-minute walking program six days per week and you will reach your target weight in no time at all.

POWER RELAXATION

Regular exercise can help to abate the mental and physical effects that stress has on your body. Under stressful conditions, your body responds by producing stress hormones (*adrenaline* and *cortisol*), as well as releasing fatty acids and glucose, which are used as fuel to produce energy. This combination of stress hormones and fuel products are the body's response to stress, known as **"fight or flight phenomena."** Both short-term stress situations and long-term stress conditions, can lead to high blood pressure, coronary artery disease, and strokes. Also, problems with digestion, headaches, anxiety, insomnia, depression, and a weakened immune system can result from long-term stress.

Physical exercise can aid the body to combat the effects of stress, by helping to burn up these stress hormones (adrenaline and cortisol) and by producing relaxing hormones called *endorphins*, which have a calming effect on the body's nervous system and help to elevate good mood feelings. Regular exercise, especially a moderate walking exercise program, helps the body combat the stress of everyday living. An aerobic exercise walking program makes you feel better and in turn helps you look better. Other relaxation activities, such as yoga and meditation, can also help you combat stress.

By combining a regular aerobic exercise walking program with strength-training exercises, using hand-held weights on the DietWalk Plan for Women, you will actually produce more endorphins (relaxation hormones), which will help your body dissipate the stress hormones (adrenalin and cortisol). This combination is one of the best methods of dealing with stress and tension. As you continue on your Power Diet-Step program, your body will continue to burn calories and increase your metabolic rate. This increased metabolic rate will boost your energy level as it decreases your stress hormones and increases your relaxation hormones. Walk away stress and tension and let the feel-good hormones wash over your body.

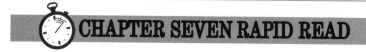

CHAPTER SEVEN RAPID READ

POWER WEIGHT-LOSS PLAN #1
(Lose one additional pound every 20 days.)

- Walk for **one hour every other day or ½ hour every day, 7 days per week.** Walking at a brisk pace of 3-3.5 mph, you will burn up approximately 350 calories every hour that you walk.

- **On this walking-off-weight Power Weight-Loss plan you will lose one additional pound every 20 days, or 1½ extra pounds every month.**

POWER WEIGHT-LOSS PLAN #2
(Lose one additional pound every 10 days.)

- Walk **one hour every day of the week.** The only difference in this plan is that you are now walking an hour every day.

- You will **lose one additional pound every 10 days.** By following this plan, you can actually **lose 3 extra pounds every month.**

3. POWER WEIGHT-LOSS PLAN #3
(Lose one additional pound every 7 days.)

- Walk for **45 minutes twice daily.** When you walk 1½ hours every day, you will burn up 525 calories each day or 3,675 calories per week. You can see that you will lose a pound a week on this plan with a few extra (175 calories) to spare.

- You may divide your 1½ hours of walking into three 30 minute sessions daily if that's more convenient. The weight-loss results will be the same. This plan will enable you to **lose one additional pound every week, or about 4 extra pounds a month.**

POWER WEIGHT-LOSS SNACK PLAN

- Eat your favorite snack food, consult Table III, and walk the number of minutes listed in order to burn up the extra calories you've cheated on.

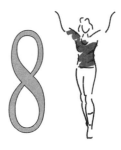

Dietwalk Body-Shaping

STRENGTH-TRAINING BURNS FAT

Studies reported at the 2014 Experimental Biology Meeting in Washington showed that short, simple, weight-training workouts helped men and women lose weight and keep that weight off permanently. Weight-training also was shown to strengthen the body's immune system, as well as lower the blood pressure. By following a low-fat, moderate protein and complex carbohydrate diet, combined with simple weight-training exercises for fourteen weeks, the participants in this study lost fat and weight, and increased the proportion of muscle to body weight. Also, these men and women showed significant improvements in blood pressure, heart rate, and aerobic fitness.

Another similar study showed that middle-aged and elderly people developed stronger muscles and a healthier immune system while walking regularly, combined with light weight-training exercises. Many of the middle-aged and elderly people in this study were moderately obese when they started the program. After twelve weeks, the majority of the obese participants had lost considerable weight, in addition to gaining lean muscle mass. These individuals also developed improved cardiovascular fitness, in addition to gaining muscle strength and boosting their energy levels.

BUILD MUSCLE MASS

Men and women after 35 to 40 years of age begin to lose muscle mass at a rate of approximately one-third pound per year. Strength training exercises makes your muscles stronger and strengthens your bones. The muscle and ligaments attached to your bones create a traction or tension on the bones when you exercise. This traction causes your bones to strengthen, by helping to absorb more calcium into the bones from the bloodstream. This process increases the mineral content of the bones, thus strengthening your bones and making them less brittle, since less calcium is lost from your bones as you age.

Aerobic exercise is great for cardiovascular fitness and burning calories, but it does not build body muscle mass. Unless we exercise, fat replaces muscle as we age. The necessity for strength training is even more pronounced in women because they begin with more fat cells and less muscle tissue compared with men. Strength training is therefore essential for weight control, strong bones and muscles, and overall fitness and well-being in everyone over the age of 35 to 40 years.

Many studies have shown that people who engage in strength training exercises develop an increase in skeletal muscle mass, whereas sedentary people lose considerable muscle mass over a period of time. Bone mineral density also increases by 1.5 % with strength-training and decreases by 2.5% in sedentary people. Also, these studies showed that strength-training in both men women increased their lean muscle mass by 4% and decreased their fat mass by 8%. This means that your muscles will become shapelier and defined and you will feel stronger because your muscles are actually stronger. You will have greater joint flexibility and have more energy when you walk. Your bones will be structurally stronger and, you will be less likely to develop osteoporosis or thinning of the bones as you get older.

Weight resistant exercises build your body's muscle mass. Improved muscle mass burns more calories by boosting your metabolism. When you build up your lean muscle mass, you can actually burn 35% more calories with exercise then you can if you were not doing strength training or strength resistance exercises. Muscle cells are more efficient at burning calories than fat cells.

On the other hand, if you just diet without exercising, you can actually lose muscle mass and subsequently decrease your basal metabolic rate. This means in effect that your basal metabolic rate slows down, so that even if you reduce your calorie intake, you will probably lose very little, if no weight at all. If you just add walking, you will increase your basal metabolic rate to five calories per minute, and if you add-strength training exercises, you will increase your basal metabolic rate to six to seven calories per minute as you build muscle mass. This is the main reason that most people who do not exercise cannot lose weight, or if they do lose weight initially, they plateau and the weight remains the same. Only by using the combination of an aerobic exercise like walking and an anaerobic exercise like strength training with hand-held weights can you actually lose weight effectively and permanently. And only then can you break through the so-called impossible plateau that happens with each and every diet.

DOUBLE BLAST OF CALORIE BURNING

Weight resistance exercises can include weight lifting, sit-ups, push-ups, aerobic exercises, swimming with flippers, skiing with poles, or walking with hand-held weights. Of all the weight-resistant exercises, walking with hand-held weights is the most efficient. That is because it combines the aerobic fitness benefits of walking with the strength training exercises of hand held weights. You have a double blast of calorie burning by walking with hand held weights. First you burn calories by the aerobic exercise of walking, and secondly, you burn additional calories by building muscles using strength training exercises. It is also the easiest type of weight training since you are not subjecting yourself to strenuous exercises or heavy weights, which can make you prone to injuries.

In addition to this double blast of calorie burning, energy boosting exercise, you get a double reward from your body. As we previously said, when you stop walking your basal metabolic rate does not decrease to the resting one calorie per minute rate. The basal metabolic rate stays at about two to three calories per minute for up to six hours after you stop walking. But now that you have added weight resistance in the form of hand held weights to walking program, you are building additional muscle mass. And as we said previously, muscle burns calories at a faster rate than fat cells and therefore you will burn additional calories after you have stopped using the hand-held weights. This means at rest, you can add another one calorie per minute burn to your walking with weights program. This translates into approximately three to four calories per minute burned when you are at rest after you have walked with hand held weights. This means that you are almost burning as many calories resting after your walk with weights as you did when you were walking without weights. It sounds impossible, doesn't it? Well, it's not! Have you ever noticed how fit, trim, muscular toned individuals can eat considerably more than unfit individuals? The reason for this is that they are always burning calories either during exercise or at rest.

WALKING WITH WEIGHTS

I usually recommend 1-pound cushioned hand-held weights, with either straps attached that go around the back of your hands, or hand-held weights with grooves for your fingers to grip the weights. After using the 1-pound weights with walking for about four to six weeks, I advise my patients to graduate to the 2-pound weights. It is important to start with one pound hand held weights and gradually build up to two pound weights after a four to six-week period. If you find that two-pound hand held weights are too heavy, then just continue your walking with weights program using one pound weights. These weights should be cushioned and covered with rubber or vinyl, since they won't rust and aren't cold to grip in cold weather. Nautilus® makes a good pair of hand-held cushioned weights with soft-foam grips and secure hand straps.

A sure-fire way to boost your calorie burning workout is to walk with hand held weights. Using hand held weights makes you work harder and improves your cardiovascular conditioning while building your upper body strength. Always check with your doctor before walking with hand held weights, especially if you have any medical condition. Also, be especially careful if you have back or joint problems before walking with hand held weights and if you find it causes any pain or discomfort, then discontinue using weights while walking.

When you start your walking with weights program, take 10 minute walks for the first 7 days so that you don't over stretch your muscles and joints. Then build up to 20 minute walks for the next 7 days. After that you can start your 30-minute walk with hand held weights two or three times a week. Initially, avoid any hills during your first six weeks while walking with hand held weights to avoid over stressing or over stretching your muscles and joints.

Do not use weighted vests around your back or chest since they will throw off your center of gravity and make walking more difficult and dangerous since you will be prone to falls and back strain. Also, avoid the use of ankle weights since they will cause you to strain your ankles and knees while walking. Injuries to these joints include ankle sprains and strains and ligament and tendon tears and cartilage injuries, especially to the knees. Ankle weights make walking difficult and strenuous and significantly increase the incidence of shin splints.

Walk with a normal arm motion as you would walk without weights. Swing your arms close to your body in a short arc. Be careful not to over-swing your arms as you can increase the risk of tendon, ligament and muscle injuries if the weights are swung in an exaggerated arc, especially above the shoulder areas. It is important to develop a walking stride and arm swing that is comfortable for you. Do not swing your arms at a greater speed than you would if you were walking naturally without weights. Also, do not swing your arms at a slower rate than you would swing than without weights because they will create a dead load on your ligaments and joints and make them prone to injury.

Walking two or three times a week is all that is necessary to build upper body strength and muscle mass. Even after you walk with weights you will continue to burn calories at a faster rate than you would if you had just walked without weights. This is because your metabolism continues to burn excessive calories even after you are finished with your exercise. Walkers burn approximately 25% more calories doing the Power Diet-Step® using handheld weights. Also, walking with weights builds lean muscle mass, which burns an additional 50 calories an hour per 1 pound of muscle. This activity is excellent for people of all ages and helps to maintain strong rotator cuff and shoulder muscles. Walking with weights also helps to develop good muscle tone, which improves balance and stability when walking. Also, walking with handheld weight helps you to develop good posture and strong chest and abdominal wall muscles.

The DIETWALK Plan is the ideal combination of an aerobic exercise, which also combines upper body strength training. There is no need to engage in strenuous aerobic exercises or to lift heavy weights at the gym (either free weights or machine weights) to achieve cardiovascular fitness, weight loss, and improved lean muscle mass. Your body will burn fat as you lose weight and you will develop a new and improved, lean and firm figure. This results from the aerobic fat-burning exercise of walking and the strength-training, muscle development of walking with weights. For people who have reached a plateau in weight loss, the ideal fat burner is pumping up your walking workouts with hand-held weights

These changes occur because of the combination of the fat-burning aerobic walking exercise and the strength-training, muscle-building exercise when you use handheld weights while walking. This is a combination that is truly impossible to reproduce. You don't have to do separate aerobic and strength-training exercises at different times or on different days. It's all combined in one easy, user-friendly exercise. Walking with weight just three days per week is all that you'll need to develop cardiovascular fitness, permanent weight loss, and a trim, slim figure. This exercise is ideal in helping to prevent osteoporosis, since walking with handheld weights puts the necessary tension on the bones and muscles, which is essential in preventing bone loss. This DIETWALK® plan is essential in helping to improve cardiovascular fitness, thus lowering blood pressure and also helping to reduce the incidence of heart disease and strokes.

DIETWALK WORKOUT

Weight resistance exercises are good for your muscles and especially good for the body's most important muscle—your heart. In a recent study by the American Heart Association, it was reported that strength training exercises can significantly lower blood pressure. Those individuals who regularly lifted light weights experienced a reduction in the systolic blood pressure (when your heart muscles contract) and a reduction in the diastolic blood pressure (when your heart muscles relax). Their resting blood pressures dropped regardless of a person's body size or weight, or whether they used heavy weight resistance exercises with longer rest periods or lighter weight exercises with shorter rest periods. In other words, using lighter weights as we suggest in the **DietWalk Walking Workout Plan,** causes the same reduction in blood pressure as those people who are lifting heavier weights. And actually, lifting heavy weights can be dangerous to your health, because over the long run they can actually raise your blood pressure. Weight resistance exercises particularly using lighter weights as in the Power Diet-Walk® Plan is safe and effective, for weight reduction and building strong bones and muscles. It's important for everyone to have a complete physical examination before using hand-held light weights in the Power Diet-Walk® Plan, especially for individuals who have had a previous heart attack, angina, high blood pressure, and irregular heart rhythm or heart valve problems.

In another recent report released by the American Heart Association, there is now increasing evidence that strength training can favorably modify many risk factors for heart disease, including blood fats (cholesterol and triglycerides), blood pressure, body fat levels and glucose metabolism. Until recently, the conventional thinking was that strength training exercises helped to build and sculpt your muscles, but did little to help the cardiovascular system and in fact, might even be harmful to your heart. This current study released by the American Heart Association dispels many of the misconceptions regarding strength training. The current study showed that strength training is beneficial using light weights for strength training.

The American Heart Association's finding in their latest study showed that weight resistance exercises should be of moderate intensity. In other words, instead of the fallacy "no pain-no gain," the truth as I've always told my patients, is "train, don't strain." The Walking Workout Plan makes your body leaner and your muscles more defined and sculptured. In addition, this plan builds stronger bones and muscles, straightens your posture, and strengthens your joints and ligaments. This plan also boosts your metabolism, which in turn helps you to lose weight. And finally, strength-training exercises enhance your sense of well-being and your self-confidence.

So, you will see that the Power Diet-Walk Walking Workout Plan not only makes you feel and look great, but helps to strengthen your heart and lower your blood pressure. In addition, it sculpts and molds your body into a figure supreme and a body that's lean. Not a bad combination for a 30-minute walking workout twice a week.

DIETWALK STEPS

No matter how long you walk, your upper body, particularly your arms, shoulders chest and upper abdomen, get a free ride. Walking is not enough to build upper body strength. Even if you pump your arms vigorously while you walk, your upper body does not get stronger because there is no resistance to encounter while you walk. On the Power Diet-Step Plan however, your legs get stronger because they encounter the resistance of the ground and thus support your body's weight. In other words, your legs get stronger, your thighs, buttocks and hips get firmer and your abdomen gets flatter on the DietWalk plan.

Weight resistance using hand-held weights while walking is a great way to put your arms to work and to strengthen your upper body muscles. This combination of walking with hand-held weights actually makes you a stronger walker. A walker's upper body should be geared towards strength and endurance, not building muscle bulk. In other words, we want to sculpt and mold the upper body (arms, back and chest). Therefore, the key to the Power Diet- Step walking workout plan is to use light-weight, hand-held weights while walking 2 or

3 days per week, while you continue your 30-minute walking plan for 6 days every week. This plan provides the unique power combination of strength training and aerobic fitness conditioning.

WILL WEIGHT TRAINING MAKE YOUR MUSCLES BULK-UP?

Many women have the misconception that weight training will result in building ugly massive muscles. Nothing could be further from the truth. In reality, women don't have to fear developing bulky muscles because of the increase in basal metabolic rate which occurs during their DietWalk strength training exercises since muscle actually burns more calories than fat; your muscles become more defined, as your muscle tissue replaces fat cells. Since women have more body fat than men, they are less likely to bulk up like men who have more muscle mass to begin with. Women will see improvement in muscle tone and strength after only 21 days on the Power Diet-Step strength training exercises. Muscles will become more defined and sculptured for a trim, firm look in both men and women. Remember this is not strenuous heavy weight lifting, this is a walking workout with light-weight, hand-held weights.

WHO BENEFITS FROM WALKING WITH WEIGHTS?

Studies reported at the 2016 Experimental Biology Meeting, showed that short, simple, weight-training workouts helped *men and women of all ages* lose weight and keep that weight off permanently. Weight-training also was shown to strengthen the body's immune system, as well as lower the blood pressure. By following a low-fat, moderate protein and complex carbohydrate diet, combined with simple weight-training exercises for fourteen weeks, the participants in this study lost fat and weight, and increased the proportion of muscle to body weight. Also, these men and women showed significant improvements in blood pressure, heart rate, and aerobic fitness.

Another similar study showed that middle-aged and elderly people developed stronger muscles and a healthier immune system while walking regularly, combined with light weight-training exercises. Many of the middle-aged and elderly people in this study were moderately obese when they started the program. After twelve weeks, the majority of the obese participants had lost considerable weight, in addition to gaining lean muscle mass. These individuals also developed improved cardiovascular fitness, in addition to gaining muscle strength and boosting their energy levels.

WHO SHOULD NOT WALK WITH WEIGHTS?

Individuals with has a medical condition such as heart or coronary artery disease. Also, people who have a neurological disorder or a degenerative or neuromuscular disease. In general, anyone who participates in the DietWalk Plan, with or without walking with weight, should first have a medical clearance from their physician.

HOW THE DIETWALK HELPS YOU LOSE WEIGHT

As you walk with light-weight, hand-held weights you build muscle mass, which in turn speeds up your metabolism. Your muscle tissue burns more calories than fat cells burn; therefore, building muscle helps to boost your resting metabolism. This increase in the resting metabolism occurs because of the actual increased muscle mass that you develop and the increased metabolic activity in the muscles themselves. By combining your 30 minutes of aerobic walking combined with strength-training exercises using hand-held weights, you have the advantage of a "power blast" of calorie burning for weight loss, while you're actually firming and toning your body's muscle mass. First of all, the aerobic walking at 3-3.5 mph in the Fit-Step® plan burns approximately 360 calories per hour or 180 calories every 30 minutes. The strength training exercises in the Power Diet-Walk® plan burn an additional 200 calories per hour or approximately 100 extra calories every 30 minutes, which is accomplished just by increasing the body's basal metabolism. So, you see you can lose more weight, more quickly by walking with hand-held weights.

IMPROVE STRENGTH AND MUSCLE TONE

The DietWalk plan is actually a walking aerobic exercise combined with an upper body strength-training exercise. As you walk with hand-held weights, you will burn an additional 25% more calories than you would burn by just walking. Walking with hand-held weights also builds lean muscle mass, which in itself burns an additional 50 calories per hour for every one pound of muscle. Walking with weights also helps to develop good muscle tone, which helps to improve balance and stability as you walk. And lastly, walking with weights also helps to develop strong arm, shoulder, chest and abdominal wall muscles, which in turn significantly improves your posture.

BOOST ENERGY AND IMPROVE FITNESS

The DietWalk is the ideal combination of an aerobic walking exercise combined with strength training using hand-held weights. It is not necessary to go to the gym in order to lift heavy weights (free weights or machine operated weights) or to engage in strenuous aerobic exercises. Just by simply walking with hand-held weights 3 days per week, you can achieve maximum cardiovascular fitness, burn calories, lose weight, and improve your lean body muscle mass. You will increase your metabolic rate as you burn fat, lose weight and boost your energy level. This combination of the aerobic fat-burning exercise of walking and the strength-training exercise of hand –held weights, is what causes you to lose weight quickly, develop a lean firm figure and develop strong bones and muscles. The DietWalk Plan is essential in helping to improve cardiovascular fitness, lower blood pressure and reduce the incidence of heart disease and strokes.

DIETWALK WORKOUTS

NATURAL ARM SWING

This is the most common arm motion that you will use naturally when walking. When you just walk without weights your arms fall into a natural, not forced, swing at the side of your body. When you walk with hand held-weights, your arms should also hang down at your side close to your body, holding the weights with your palms facing your body. As you walk, alternately swing your arms gently, as you bend your elbows ever so slightly. This is the natural arm swing motion of walking that you will be using all of the time during your regular 6 day per week 30-minute DietWalk® walking plan. This is a natural arm swing that is a motion that is most comfortable for you. Using the hand-held weights with this simple arm swing motion strengthens your triceps and upper shoulder muscles.

LOCOMOTIVE ARM MOTION

This is the arm motion that you see runners or fast walkers use while they are running or walking fast. Hold your arms close to your body and bend your arms at approximately a 90-degree angle at the elbow, so the that your hands are making a slight fist facing in front of you. Hold the weights with palms facing your body. Now, do the locomotive! Start to move your arms alternately forward and backward. This motion strengthens the muscles of your upper arm, triceps and shoulder muscles.

Just do this exercise for a few minutes at a time during your 30-minute walk and the go back to the natural arm swing. You can increase the number of minutes that you do the Locomotive Arm Motion as you develop more upper body strength, after you've been walking with weights for several weeks. Do not continue with this exercise if it initially causes muscle strain or pain. If you just work into it very gently, you will be able to build upper body strength gradually on the DietWalk plan.

HAMMER CURL SWING

This exercise begins exactly like the first natural arm swing exercise. Keep your arms hanging down at your sides close to your body, holding the weights with your palms facing your body. As you walk, bend each arm alternately at the elbow, towards your shoulder, and then lower each arm to the side of your body. Be sure to keep your arms close to your body. Pretend you're hammering a nail into a piece of wood or banging your fists on to a table top. This exercise strengthens your forearm and biceps muscles.

It is important to only do this exercise for a few minutes at a time during your 30-minute walk and gradually build up the number of minutes using the Hammer Curl as you slowly improve your upper body strength over a period of many weeks on the Power Diet-Step plan. Remember to revert to the Natural Arm Swing motion when you stop the Hammer Curl. Also, discontinue this exercise if it causes any pain or strain on your muscles and try it again at a later date.

This exercise is much safer to do while walking than is the traditional biceps curl, where your palms face away from your body and your wrists are rotated outward. You will prevent the hand-held weights from bumping your legs as you walk when you do the hammer curl instead of the traditional biceps curl. Also, you get better muscle strengthening and toning with this exercise.

MORE ADVANCED WALKING WORKOUTS

The previous three exercises are the basic walking with weights exercises. Once you've become comfortable with these three exercises say after 4-6 weeks, you can then begin to try the more advanced walking with hand-held weights exercises. If these appear too difficult or strenuous to do while you're walking, then do them at the end of your 30-minute walk, when you are standing still.

REACH FOR THE SKY

Bend your arms at the side of your body with your elbows bent and pointing towards your feet. Hold the weights in your hands, palms facing your body at shoulder level. Do not turn your wrists outwards as weight-lifters do when they lift heavy weights. Raise the weights above head, until arms are fully extended. Then lower weights back down to shoulder level. Again, do this exercise for only a few minutes at a time during your 30-minute walking workout. This exercise can slowly be increased as you continue to build upper body strength over a period of many weeks on the DietWalk plan. Again, remember to discontinue the Reach for the Sky exercise if it causes pain or strain in your muscles.

Now, reach for the sky! Think of this exercise as lifting the weight of the world off of your shoulders as you reach for the sky. This exercise sculpts and strengthens the upper back and shoulder muscles.

Flap Your Wings

Hold the weights next to the sides of your legs, palms facing in. Lift both arms together, out to your sides and away from your body. Lift arms out away from your body, to just slightly below the level of your shoulders (no higher) as you walk, and then lower both arms to your sides. This exercise must be done carefully while you're walking; otherwise you may lose your balance or knock into someone or something that is next to you while you're walking. Remember to only do this exercise for a few minutes at a time and then revert to the Natural Arm Swing motion for the rest of your 30- minute Power Diet-Step walk. If you find that this exercise is too difficult to do while walking, then wait until your walk is finished and then do 10-12 repetitions of the Flap Your Wings exercise. This exercise strengthens your upper back, chest and shoulder muscles.

Butterfly Stroke

Hold weights in each hand in front of you at chest level, palms facing each other and your elbows bent at 90 degrees pointing towards your feet. Spread both arms out to your sides like a butterfly, being careful not to spread your arms out too wide past your shoulder level. Then bring the weights back together in front of you at chest level. Be careful not to bang your hands or the weights together. You can also vary this exercise by extending your arms directly in front of you and then spread your arms out to your sides and then bring them back together. Only do this exercise for a few minutes if you try it while walking and then revert to the Natural Arm Swing motion for the rest of your 30-minute walk. As with the other exercises, stop this one also if you feel pain or strain in your muscles. As you gradually build up your upper body strength you can try this exercise slowly and gently during or after your 30-minute walk.

This exercise is particularly good for strengthening, developing and sculpting mid-chest and upper back muscles.

If you find this exercise is too difficult to do while walking, then you can do it at the end of your 30-minute walk. If you're tired, you can even do this exercise lying down as follows:

1. Lie on your back, with your knees bent and your feet flat on the floor.

2. Start with arms stretched out above you towards the ceiling with weights in each hand, with palms facing each other.

3. Slowly lower your arms out to the sides, and then gently pull arms back to starting positions directly above and in front of you. Use primarily your chest muscles while doing this exercise, not your arm muscles.

DIETWALK WORKOUT EXERCISE TIPS

Start with 1-pound weights in each hand for the first 4 weeks, and then you can build up to 2-pound weights after you feel comfortable walking with 1-pound weights. If you find however, that 2-pound weights are too heavy, then stick with the 1-pound weights. Studies show that you still will get the same great muscle strengthening, toning and sculpting with very light weights. Actually, most people do just fine with one pound weights.

The DietWalk Exercises only have to be done 3 days per week to achieve maximum strength training and muscle toning benefits. If the weather is bad, then these exercises can be done at home. Only do one set of 10-12 repetitions of each exercise after your 30-minute indoor workout. After you've been doing these exercises for 21 days, then you can build up to two or three sets of 10-12 repetitions per week for increased calorie burning and improved muscle tone.

Only try the advanced exercises when you've become thoroughly conditioned, after you've completed 21-days on the DietWalk plan. You can vary the exercises as you walk. Remember to stop any particular DietWalk exercise if you become tired or your muscles become sore of feel stained. Remember, these exercises can be done at the end of your 30-minute walk, if you find them too difficult to do while walking. Start with one set of 10-12 repetitions of each exercise at the end of your walk and then you can build them up to two or three sets of 10-12 repetitions after you've completed the first 21-days of your DietWalk walking plan.

Tighten your abdominal muscles intermittently while you're doing these exercises, whether you're walking or standing still at the time. This helps to provide support for your upper body and back, while helping to trim, tone and flatten your abdominal muscles.

How would you like to lighten your load as you continue on your DietWalk 30- minute walk? Instead of using hand-held weights, you can occasionally carry one 24- ounce plastic bottle of water in each hand. As you proceed on your 30-minute walk, you can drink from each bottle alternately, until each bottle becomes lighter and lighter. When you're finished with your workout, you will be refreshed and rehydrated

HOW MANY REPETITIONS SHOULD YOU DO WITH EACH EXERCISE?

You'll be able to customize the number of repetitions for each exercise depending on your own comfort level. During the first 21-days on the DietWalk Plan it's only necessary to do one set of 10-12 repetitions for each exercise. This is usually adequate strength training, as you rotate from one exercise to another. Then you should revert to your Natural Arm Swing motion of walking for the rest of your 30-minute walk. Remember to start slowly with fewer repetitions when you start your walking workout and gradually build up the number of repetitions until you reach your own comfort level.

ONCE YOU'RE FIT, IT TAKES LONGER TO GET OUT OF SHAPE

What if I can't keep up with the exercise plan regularly? What if I have to stop for a few days or a week or even longer if some interruption in my life prevents me from continuing? This is the kind of thinking that prevents many men and women from starting an exercise program and prevents others from going back to one that they've already begun. Never fear, the answer's here—*"It takes much longer to get out of shape than it does to get into shape."*

The DietWalk is forgiving. Even if you miss a few days or a week or a few weeks in a month, there is no need to worry. Once you have been conditioned physically, it takes a lot longer to get out of shape than it took you to get into shape. The rate of regression depends on how long you've been exercising and how fit you are. The body is remarkable, since it tends to hold on to these fitness gains long after you've stopped exercising. Most women lose muscle strength at about at about one-half the rate at which they gained it. So, if you've been doing the DietWalk Plan for three months, and have to discontinue for any reason, it could take up to six months for your body to fall back to its pre-training state.

Aerobic capacity starts to decrease in the first two to three weeks after you've stopped exercising, but it can take almost six to eight months before fit exercisers get back to the fitness level where they started. Aerobic exercising (walking) decreases the LDL (bad cholesterol) and increases the HDL (good cholesterol) after you've been on your walking program for approximately two to three weeks after you've stopped exercising, but it can take almost six to eight months before fit exercisers get back to the fitness level where they started. Aerobic exercising (walking) decreases the LDL (bad cholesterol) and increases the HDL (good cholesterol) after you've been on your walking program for approximately two to three months. Studies show that it took at least three months for these cholesterol levels to return to their original pre-walking workout levels after the exercise of walking was discontinued.

That's pretty good, considering you've stopped walking all that time. When walkers resume their walking program, it took them only one-half the time to return to their original levels of fitness. So, don't worry if you have to discontinue your walking program for any reason or for any period of time. The benefits that you've worked so hard for are long lasting and they are easily obtained again in one half the time. **The DietWalk is forgiving and it keeps on giving!**

CHAPTER EIGHT RAPID READ

- Short, simple, weight-training workouts helped men and women lose weight and keep that weight off permanently.

- Strength training exercises makes your muscles stronger and strengthens your bones.

- Walking with hand-held weights is the most efficient. That is because it combines the aerobic fitness benefits of walking with the strength training exercises of hand held weights.

- Walking with 1- or 2-pound weights improves your cardiovascular conditioning while building your upper body strength

- Walking two or three times a week is all that is necessary to build upper body strength and muscle mass.

- Muscle tissue burns more calories than fat cells burn; therefore, building muscle helps to boost your resting metabolism.

- Strength-training exercises you can do while walking include:
  - Natural Arm Swing
  - Locomotive Arm Motion
  - Hammer Curl Swing
  - Reach for the Sky
  - Flap Your Wings
  - Butterfly Stroke

- Most women lose muscle strength at about at about one-half the rate at which they gained it.

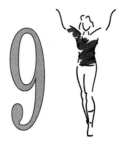

Look Younger & Live Longer!

The facts are irrefutable: you live longer and have an improved quality of life if you're a walker. Recent medical studies indicate that women walkers live at least 10-15 years longer than non-walkers, and in many cases, up to 20 years longer.

In a recent study conducted on over 20,000 college graduates, it was determined that those women who exercised regularly lived significantly longer than those who remained sedentary. The women who exercised consistently had a significantly lower incidence of heart attacks and strokes than those in the sedentary group. And the exercise that most of these graduates reported was—*walking.* Those who walked the most had the lowest incidence of early death. The individuals who walked 9-10 miles per week (that's only about 20 minutes daily or 40 minutes every other day) had a 20% lower risk of heart attacks than those who walked 2-3 miles per week, and a 30% lower risk than those who didn't walk at all. Walking adds years to your life and life to your years. *Walk as if your life depended on it*—It Does!

FEEL & LOOK YOUNGER

Walking produces a remarkable number of changes that occur inside of your body. Your blood volume and the red blood cells increase in number. Your *heart* pumps blood more efficiently. Your *lungs* expand, taking in and distributing more oxygen. Your *muscles* tighten and contract giving you a firmer figure. Your *energy level* increases, and you feel strong and fit. The results of these changes will make your figure lean and your posture supreme.

Your overall appearance will improve following your daily walk, since walking will improve your circulation and enable you to feel and look great. Your skin, complexion, and hair texture will also improve with walking because of the increased blood circulation to the skin and hair follicles. Your complexion will literally glow after your walk and your skin will stay healthy and fresh looking all day long.

After you have been walking for a while you will notice that your muscles will become firm and many of the fatty deposits on your thighs and buttocks will start to decrease in size. Your stomach will become flatter and the muscles of your calves, thighs, and buttocks will become firmer and shapelier. These changes result from improved muscle tone and also from the strengthening of muscles and ligaments, which are attached to the spine.

You don't have to kill yourself to stay fit, trim, and healthy. Walking actually provides better long-term figure control and fitness benefits than jogging or other strenuous exercises, without the hazards and dangers. Always remember that exercise does not have to be painful or uncomfortable to be effective. The DIETWALK Plan, consists of walking for 30 minutes, 6 days per week, and walking for 30 minutes using light, hand-held weights for 3 days per week, provides the easy steps needed for a trim, beautiful body.

BE WONDER WOMAN

Just think how many hours a day we waste in front of our TV sets. Or how many hours we sit at our desks and work every day. Consider the number of hours that we spend inside of our cars daily, going from here to there and everywhere. And what about our free time? Do we ever go out for a walk? Do we spend any time moving our sedentary bodies? No, we just log on to the Internet, and spend hour after hour looking for anything and everything that in reality is "much ado about nothing." And no matter how you put it, all we do is "**just sit there.**" Is it any wonder that we are an overweight, under-exercised society? Can there be any doubt "just sitting there" is a major cause of a number of diseases, disability, and even premature death? We have been raised in the "just sitting there" mode, in part caused by the advances in technology, which leaves us very little to do that actually involves physical motion of any kind.

I know many of you at one time or another have joined a gym and made a real effort at exercise. But most of you have found that the time involved and the strenuous effort required only leads to frustration and ennui. After working all day, how can anyone keep up with the bionic, 20-year-old, aerobics instructor? How can anyone continuously hop from machine to endless machine, so that each and every tiny muscle in our bodies is exercised to the maximum? Who in their right mind would attempt to lift weights that even Hercules would find difficult? And how can anyone after a long hard day at work, muster up the strength to run and run and even run faster on the mechanical motion monster machines that send our hearts pumping ever so fast, our blood pressure rising precipitously, and our muscles, ligaments and joints screaming "pain, pain, pain?" Is it any wonder why most of us finally give up our home exercise programs or our fitness club memberships, so that we can finally do what we have been genetically programmed to do all of our lives. "Let's just sit there. We really need our rest. I just don't have the time to exercise or work out. Those exercise machines were far too formidable and powerful for the likes of us. Yes, we concede the fact that the machines have won. Let's just sit there and rest."

Well, let's not get too comfortable yet. We don't have to "just sit there." Even though the machines have beaten us, we can take heart in the fact that we are still alive, albeit maimed and weakened. And would you believe it, the machines don't even have as much as a scratch on them. But take heart, my fellow exercisers: you actually have your own secret machine built into your mortal bodies. This machine will not harm or injure you. This machine will not break your bones and limbs. This machine will not elevate your blood pressure and heart rate to dangerous levels. This is your very own personal body machine that has been with you all of your lives, and very few of you know of its power and its benefits. Yes, this machine is made up of your blood and your heart and your ligaments and joints and your muscles and bones and the rest of your wonderful anatomy. **It's your very own friendly walking machine.** It's been there forever, and for whatever reason it has been gathering dust in the cobwebs of your mind. You have never even considered what a powerful and awesome machine your walking machine can be.

To walk is akin to breathing. To walk is what helps your life's blood circulate and provide oxygen to all of your body's cells. Walking aids in your digestion, in your metabolism, and in your breathing and circulation. Walking helps to lubricate and strengthen your muscles, joints, and ligaments. Walking helps your heart to stay healthy, and walking supplies oxygen and nutrients to all of your body's cells. Walking keeps your brain supplied with oxygen so that you can finally realize what a powerful machine you had hidden away somewhere in the recesses of your brain and walking is the secret code that can be used to overcome our genetic predisposition to "just sit there." By walking, we override the synapses in our brains that tell us that we should "just be sitting there." We actually now have the scientific technology to reprogram our "just-sitting- there-genes," and in a sense, alter our DNA. Now we will be able to get out of our chairs, out of our cars, out from in front of our computers and TVs, and propel us forward so that we can now move about freely without supervision or restriction. And then we can finally say, "Yes, I really can lose 12 pounds in two weeks, and become fit in spite of myself."

EAT LESS—LIVE MORE

Reducing your daily calorie intake by just 20-25% daily can extend your life by 10-15 years, according to a recent study released by the National Center for Toxicological Research. Based on animal studies, their findings regarding decreased calorie consumption were as follows:

- Extends life and delays the aging process by enhancing DNA'S ability to repair cell damage that results in disease and aging.

- Slows or prevents cancer by making the metabolism more efficient in eliminating carcinogens from the body.

- Slows the metabolic rate and lowers the body temperature, which in turn slows the aging process.

These findings are based on studies which appear to delay the aging process by reducing both the total daily caloric intake and the intake of total fats in the diet. It is essential to provide adequate vitamins, minerals and nutrients in a calorie reduced diet in order to slow the aging process. There must also be a balance between the intake of proteins, carbohydrates and fats.

Women who walk regularly are usually not big eaters. Perhaps that fact combined with the life-extension benefits of walking is what accounts for the very long life spans of walkers. *Eating less and walking more will give you a long-life for evermore!*

MYSTERY OF THE AGING PROCESS

Modern medical research is constantly probing the mysteries of the aging process. Molecular biology and genetic engineering are two of the important tools being used by today's scientists in their effort to unravel the complex changes that accompany aging. Since the National Institute on Aging was founded in 1975, research funding has gone from approximately 15 million dollars to over 400 million dollars in 2015.

The average life expectancy for men is 76.5 years and for women 83.2 years. Many scientists believe that the life span could easily be extended to well over 100 years if some of the mysteries of the aging process are decoded. After the age of 28-32, the aging process begins to "kick in." These changes first begin at the molecular level in all of the body's cells from the tiniest organs like the parathyroid and pituitary glands to the largest organs like the liver and skin.

Molecular genetics has found that each animal species has a different lifespan, including humans. So, what's a body to do? Many people take the fatalistic attitude that their genes will determine when they are to die and that nothing whatsoever can be done to change their genetic code. Nothing could be further from the truth. There are a number of factors that affect the body's *immune system,* which in turn affects the body's ability to repair damaged or degenerated genes. If, in fact, we can alter the genetic code in a somewhat similar fashion to what scientists do in genetic engineering, then we could conceivably alter life expectancy.

Well, you can do just that! You can **live longer and look younger**. You can modify or alter your genetic code and beat the odds against dying an early death or a predetermined genetic-coded death for that matter. The following secrets for breaking the genetic code and beefing up your immune system are:

BREAK THE GENETIC CODE

Stress produces the release of the hormones **adrenalin** and **glucocorticoids** produced by the adrenal glands. High levels of these chemicals accelerate the aging process by speeding up the death of tiny brain cells and they damage nerve cells throughout the body. These two hormones also produce molecules called *free-radicals* that contain a very reactive form of oxygen. These free-radicals can damage the heart, blood vessels, and the lining of the lungs. They also have been implicated in the development of certain forms of cancer and arthritis.

Well, how do you avoid stress? It's not as easy as it sounds, is it? Actually, it really is. The first thing you have to be aware of is that *stress always wins—if you let it.* The way not to let stress win is to beat it at its own game. Stress has a lot of henchmen on its side—adrenalin, glucocorticoids, and free-radicals. Well, who do you have on your side, willing to back you up every step of the way? *Your feet*—that's who! Those two little fellows can beat any adrenalin, glucocorticoids, and free radicals twice their size.

First of all, when confronted with stress, say the magic words: **feet retreat!** No one alive or dead for that matter has ever beat stress standing toe-to-toe. If you make the mistaken decision to fight it out with stress, be prepared to go down for the count of ten and then some—maybe forever! Stress always wins when you confront it head on. The reason is that stress's henchmen—adrenalin, glucocorticoids, and free-radicals have a 1-2-3 punch that's impossible to beat.

Adrenalin speeds up your heart rate and squeezes your blood vessels shut. It causes your pupils to dilate and your skin to become cold and clammy. It shuts down your kidneys and speeds up your intestinal tract. It elevates your blood pressure to dangerous levels making the possibility of a stroke or heart attack likely. Can you beat that first punch? Not if your life depended on it!

Glucocorticoids also narrow down your blood vessels and speed up your heart rate. They cause your body to retain liquid, which can lead to heart failure. They also cause sodium retention from your kidneys, which can further elevate your blood pressure to dangerous levels. They can also damage your kidneys and the adrenal glands themselves, which actually produced the glucocorticoids in the first place. And lastly, they have an adverse effect on your pancreas and can lead to an over-production of insulin, which results in sharp rises and falls in your blood glucose levels—not a good thing at all for your overall health. Think you can duck that number two punch? Not in a million years!

And what about that last punch—**free radicals**. Free radicals are maverick atoms of oxygen that are produced by the stress reaction. They can cause the deterioration of blood vessels and the alveoli (tissues that line the lungs). They can damage the heart by causing degeneration of the heart tissue. These free radicals, and they really are radical, can cause a decrease in the regular oxygen supply to all of the body's cells and tissues including the heart muscle itself. Without oxygen, organs and tissues die. Without oxygen, heart muscle and brain cells die. These nutty hyped-up oxygen atoms can even cause glaucoma, arthritis, and nerve damage. Don't even try to think about beating these crazy little atoms, you'd lose every time.

So, what about that secret ingredient I spoke about earlier? **Feet Retreat!** The only way to beat these stress factors (adrenalin, glucocorticoids, and free radicals) is to turn on your heels and beat a quick retreat. *Walking away from stress* is your only defense against these dangerous destroyers. Walking away actually dissipates these three killers from your bloodstream. As you walk the levels of adrenalin, glucocorticoids, and free radicals start to decline. The relaxation hormones-beta-endorphins start to permeate your tissues and cells while the three killer chemicals are pushed out of your bloodstream and eliminated from the body by your liver and kidneys.

Stress is actually a state of mind and if you're willing to succumb to it, you will. If you learn relaxation techniques, walking being the main one, you will learn to deal with stress effectively, rather than letting stress deal effectively with you. A refreshing walk not only dissipates the stress chemicals from the body but it also dissipates the negative thought processes from the brain. It clears the cobwebs and sweeps the dust out of the corners of your mind. It scrubs clean the walls of your aggressiveness and intolerance. It cleanses the windows of your intellect and it sharpens your mental awareness and understanding, so that you can deal with stress intellectually rather than emotionally. Yes, walking does all that and then some—try it! It works! Here's a prime example of walking to win, and winning here is more than just winning—it's your life. You can beat stress from within if you follow the DIETWALK Plan.

BEEF UP YOUR IMMUNE SYSTEM

It's important to select foods that are high in minerals and vitamins and low in fats and reined sugars. Eat more fruit, vegetables, fowl, and fish and less meat and dairy products.

Foods high in saturated fats are particularly harmful to the immune system. These foods raise blood cholesterol levels which clog the arteries and subsequently slow down the flow of oxygen-rich blood and vital nutrients to the body's cells and tissues.

This process actually shortens your life expectancy by allowing your vital organs and tissues to die a slow, painful death. No organ can live without adequate supplies of oxygen and nutrients. High-fat foods also take considerably longer than other foods to convert to energy. Eating a high-fat meal diverts blood and oxygen from the brain to the digestive tract, leaving you feeling fatigued and light-headed.

Blood cholesterol levels can also be lowered by eating more fruits, vegetables, fowl, and fish and reducing consumption of meats, dairy products, and pastries, especially those made with palm or coconut oil. The fiber in beans, legumes, and oat bran lowers cholesterol as well as the pectin in fruits such as apples, oranges, and grapefruit.

Refined sugar plays havoc with the immune system by triggering sudden rises in insulin production which result in dramatic sharp drops in blood glucose levels. This condition known as hypoglycemia can result in fatigue, headaches, fainting spells, weakness, and even convulsions. Not only is the body deprived of essential glucose for energy and metabolism, but the brain is also deprived of essential glucose, which is necessary for brain function. If the brain cells are deprived of glucose for any length of time, then some of these brain cells may atrophy or die.

Like oxygen, these brain cells need a constant infusion of glucose to enable the neurological network to function properly. Once deprived of glucose, the brain exhibits memory loss, loss of coordination, speech impairment, generalized muscle weakness, and even convulsions if glucose deprivation persists for a long period of time.

VITAMINS AND MINERALS FOR HEALTH

Remember when we spoke about the arch villains called the free radicals? Well, a diet high in yellow and dark green vegetables provides *Beta-carotene,* which is a precursor to vitamin A. This chemical Beta-carotene breaks up free radicals and protects the body against their harmful effects such as cancer and degenerative diseases. Likewise, vitamin E found in many cereal grains, fish, and non-fat dairy products also protects against the villainous free radicals. An adequate supply of vitamins C and B-complex are essential to keep the immune system in good working order. These water-soluble vitamins are essential for good health and longevity.

Fruits and vegetables provide an excellent source of these vitamins, but they must be continuously supplied to the body. Being water-soluble, they are excreted rapidly. A daily vitamin supplement of B complex and vitamin C is recommended to keep the body's cells and tissues constantly supplied with these essential vitamins. These vitamins are responsible for keeping the immune system in good working order and they help the body to repair its own DNA (the material that makes up your genes).

AVOID STRESS AND SLEEP WELL

SLEEP

Most people require between 6-8 hours of sleep per night. Some individuals need less, others need more. If you wake refreshed in the morning and don't tire easily during the day, then you're probably getting enough sleep. The sleep/wake cycle is affected by many things; one in particular is the release of a hormone called cortisol. This hormone decreases before bedtime and starts to rise in the early morning hours before you wake. Travel and shift-work can affect your sleeping cycle by interfering with the cortisol blood levels. Your body usually will adjust to time changes after several days, by changing the rise and fall of cortical production.

There is also a condition which is usually caused by stress, called night-eating disorder syndrome or NES, which is actually an eating disorder. People with NES wake up several times during the night and are unable to fall back to sleep unless they eat something, usually high-fat, high-sugar junk foods. Unfortunately, they are often awakened again by the subsequent drop in blood sugar level that makes them hungry again. The best remedy for this condition is for the person with this particular sleep disorder, is to have a small portion of a lean, high- protein snack. For example, a slice of low-fat cheese, a handful of nuts, nonfat yogurt, a glass of skim or soy milk or even a slice of low fat turkey will usually satisfy that night-time hunger. These lean, high-protein. snacks are appetite satisfying, take longer to digest than carbohydrates, and help break the vicious junk-food binge-eating cycle of night-time eating.

KEEP MENTALLY ACTIVE

As you age you can expect fatigue and a dulling of the mental senses unless you keep mentally active. Keeping mentally active requires that you continuously stimulate the brain cells by reading, doing puzzles, playing games such as checkers, chess, or cards, keeping up with or learning a new hobby or skill, or constantly interacting with other people. By keeping mentally alert you will stay younger longer and enjoy your years with less fatigue and more energy and pep. Remember, it's important to think young! Staying young is as much a state of mind as it is a state of body physiology.

STOP SEDENTARY SITTING

Inactivity is associated with obesity, diabetes, hypertension, heart disease, pulmonary and gastrointestinal disorders, arthritis, back problems, muscular and mental tension, and premature death. Walking, on the other hand, increases the delivery of oxygen to the brain and body tissues, which improves the circulation. This results in increased energy and mental alertness. Walking also decreases stress and tension thus producing muscular and mental relaxation. This in turn lowers the blood pressure and prevents cardiovascular disease. Walking also lowers the LDL-bad cholesterol and raises HDL-good cholesterol, protecting you from heart disease.

Walking burns calories and prevents or controls obesity and diabetes. Walking builds muscle and bone tissue and prevents osteoporosis, arthritis, and degenerative muscular and back disorders. Walking prevents the development of chronic lung disorders by keeping the lungs and respiratory muscles in good working order and by preventing the lung capacity from shrinking.

Walking boosts the immune system by producing chemicals known as **interferons** that do everything from warding off colds to preventing cancer. In fact, when you come right down to it, walking prevents almost every known disease and disability known to modern science. And above all, walking prevents premature death and even mature death. Walking will allow you to live years beyond your pre-determined genetic-code death. Population studies show that *walkers live at least 15-20 years longer* than their sedentary counterparts.

STEPS TO A LONG LIFE

How long you live depends partly on your genetic code. Heredity does play an important role in your longevity factor. However, you can beat your genetic code if you eliminate most of the risk factors of heart disease, hypertension, vascular disease, and cancer. The following simplified list is an outline of what you can do to eliminate many of the risk factors that are present in our everyday lives. **Here are 12 steps to a longer life:**

1. Decrease salt intake and you help to prevent or lessen the risk of hypertension and stroke.

2. Maintain normal weight to prevent the risk of hypertension, heart disease, obesity, and diabetes.

3. Decrease cholesterol in the diet to lessen the chance of heart attacks, strokes, and blood clots.

4. Decrease saturated fat in the diet to lower blood cholesterol in order to prevent strokes and heart attacks, and to lessen the risk of breast, prostate, and colon cancer.

5. Increase the fiber in your diet to lower cholesterol and to prevent the development of hemorrhoids, varicose veins, diverticulitis, and colon cancer.

6. Increase consumption of green and yellow vegetables, which have high concentrations of vitamin A & C, to prevent various types of intestinal cancer.

7. Avoid the use of smoked-meats and smoked-fishes, which have high concentrations of nitrites that lead to stomach and esophageal cancer.

8. Avoid the use of excess caffeine, which can lead to breast cysts, breast cancer, pancreatic cancer, prostate cancer, nervous disorders, heart disease, and high blood pressure.

9. Avoid the use of tobacco, which can cause oral cancer, lung cancer, emphysema, hypertension, and heart disease.

10. Avoid excess alcohol consumption, which may contribute to liver cirrhosis, liver cancer, hepatitis, pancreatic tumors, heart disease, and neurological disorders.

11. Avoid prolonged exposure to the sun to prevent the development of skin cancer.

12. Avoid stress whenever possible to prevent the body's stress hormones from raising your blood pressure and constricting your arteries.

IMPROVE CELLULAR OXYGEN

In addition to these twelve steps, make sure that you have regular check-ups with your family physician. Be sure to carefully follow any recommendations that s/he has as to your diet, exercise, medications, etc. If you're ever in doubt as to your doctor's advice, don't hesitate to get a second opinion. The worst thing that you can do is to ignore your doctor's recommendations. Also, never be afraid to ask him or her questions about things that bother you. And never, ever ignore any unusual signs or symptoms that you develop. Check with your doctor immediately. Don't hide your head in the sand like an ostrich, hoping that these symptoms or signs will go away by themselves.

There is no segment of the population that could benefit more from a walking program than the elderly. A younger person can increase his/her physical fitness 15-25% by exercising, an older person may be able to improve his or her physical fitness 35-50%. As our population gets older, more people are realizing the benefits of regular moderate exercise. A recent national poll found that over 50% of women 65 and older walk regularly every day.

Walking can reverse or slow down the ravages of the aging process as we have previously seen. Walking helps to control weight, lower blood cholesterol, and decrease body fat. Walking helps to build bone structure, strengthen ligaments and tendons, and increase muscle mass and strengthen muscle tissue. Walking helps to condition the lungs and respiratory muscles and improves the general overall breathing capacity. Walking also helps the cardiovascular and circulatory systems by improving the efficiency of the heart's pumping action. Walking helps to keep the blood vessels elastic, preventing the development of hypertension. Walking keeps the blood circulating and prevents the formation of blood clots by preventing the blood platelets from sticking together.

And finally, walking helps to improve the maximum oxygen uptake, which increases the oxygen uptake from the atmosphere, its distribution through the bloodstream and its final delivery to the cells of the body's organs and tissues. *This improved oxygenation at the cellular level is the basis for the life process itself.* If you can provide a constant infusion of oxygen on a regular basis at the cellular level, then you can slow down the aging process. By providing this oxygen to the cells, your body can operate its cellular machinery more efficiently. The body's cells can utilize the nutrients they receive from the bloodstream more efficiently when they are saturated with oxygen.

SHAPE-UP & BE YOUNG

1. **Walking lowers the blood pressure by:**

   A. dilating (opening) the arteries, allowing more blood to flow through them

   B. improving elasticity of blood vessels-giving less resistance to the flow of blood

   C. lowering chemicals in blood that can raise blood pressure-catecholamines and angiotensin

D. improving return of blood to the heart, so that the heart can work more efficiently at a slower rate

E. increasing the amount of oxygen delivered to all tissues and cells

F. decreasing the rate of sodium reabsorption in the kidneys

2. Walking protects the heart by:

A. decreasing the risk of blood clot formation

B. improving the return of blood to the heart from the leg veins

C. increasing the flow of blood through the coronary arteries

D. increasing HDL (good) cholesterol, which protects the heart and arteries against fatty deposits (plaque)

E. improving the efficiency of the heart's cardiac output (total volume of blood pumped out by the heart each minute)

F. helping to keep the collateral circulation open and available for emergencies

3. Walking improves lung efficiency and breathing capacity by:

A. conditioning the muscles of respiration (chest wall and diaphragm)

B. opening more usable lung space (alveoli)

C improving efficiency of extracting oxygen from the air

4. Walking improves the general circulation by:

A. increasing the total volume of blood, and the amount of red blood cells, allowing more oxygen to be carried in the bloodstream

B. dilating the arteries, thus improving blood flow

C. increasing flexibility of arteries, thus lowering blood pressure

D. compression of leg and abdominal veins by the pumping action of the muscles used in walking, aiding the return of blood to the heart

E. using small blood vessels in the legs for rerouting blood (collateral circulation) around blocked arteries in emergencies

5. Walking prevents the build-up of fatty deposits (plaque) in arteries by:

A. decreasing the serum triglycerides (sugar fats)

B. decreasing LDL (bad) cholesterol in the blood

C. increasing HDL (good) cholesterol in the blood

D. preventing the blood from getting too thick, thus lessening the chance that blood clots will form

6. Walking promotes weight loss and weight control by:

A. directly burning calories

B. regulating the brain center (appestat) to control appetite

C. redirecting blood flow away from digestive tract toward the exercising muscles, thus decreasing appetite

D. using blood fats instead of sugar as a source of energy

7. Walking controls stress by:

A. increasing relaxation hormones in the brain (Beta-endorphins) and decreasing stress hormones (epinephrine and norepinephrine)

B. increasing the oxygen supply and decreasing the amount of carbon dioxide to the brain

C. efficiently utilizing blood sugar in the body regulated by an improved production of insulin

D. literally walking away from stress

8. Walking promotes a longer healthier life by:

A. strengthening the heart muscle and regulating the cardiac output (a slower more efficient heart rate)

B. lowering blood pressure, thus preventing strokes, heart attacks and kidney disorders

C. improving lungs' efficiency in extracting oxygen from air

D. improving the efficiency of the delivery of oxygen to all the body's organs, tissues, and cells

E. strengthening muscle fibers throughout the body thus improving reaction time and maintaining muscle tone

F. maintaining bone strength and structure by preserving the mineral content of the bone, thus preventing osteoporosis (bone thinning) and certain forms of osteoporosis.

WOMEN WALKERS WIN

As the organs and tissues of the body age, they become susceptible to the ravages of disease, illness, and cancer. The aging cells of the various organs and tissues of the body break down gradually, losing the ability to operate their internal metabolic machinery properly. Viral infections, bacterial infections, degenerative diseases, and cancer cells can invade these weakened cells of your body, as these cells go through the aging process.

The list of degenerative changes that occurs in every living cell in your body as you age can be slowed down! That gradual decrease in both mental and physical functions can be reversed! Those aging organs, tissues, and cells can be given new life again! No, you can't prevent the aging process from proceeding, but you certainly can slow down its progress to a snail's crawl.

You can stand up and take charge of your life and prevent the degenerative ravages of aging from crumbling your body like an old building. There is a way for you to *reverse the aging process* **and** *add years to your life.* Yes, the answer is **WALKING. Walk as if your life depended on it—It Does!**

Women walkers by and large live at least 15 years longer than sedentary women. Walkers in every country in the world have been proven to be the longest-living segment of any population of civilization. From the Masii natives in Africa to the Russian tribes in Siberia; from the mountain climbers of Peru to the Bushman of New Guinea; from the hikers in Ireland to the mail carriers of the United States. All of these people have one thing in common—*they're all walkers!* And for all intents and purposes they live longer than any other similar-age group of sedentary people in their respective cities or countries.

Dr. Alexander Leaf, chairman Dept. of Preventive Medicine, Massachusetts General Hospital, studied various populations throughout the world and concluded that the active segment of each population lived considerably longer than the inactive segment. He stated, *"It is apparent that an exercise like walking throughout life is an important factor promoting well-being and longevity. One is never too old to commence a regular program of exercise and once started, will never grow too old to continue it."* Walkers live longer and are illness-free longer than their sedentary counterparts anywhere in the world. This was the conclusion reached at the last national convention on *Clinical Research on Aging.*

CHAPTER NINE RAPID READ

- Women walkers live at least 10-15 years longer than non-walkers, and in many cases, up to 20 years longer.

- Walking aids in your digestion, metabolism, and breathing and circulation. Walking helps lubricate and strengthen your muscles, joints, and ligaments. Walking helps your heart to stay healthy, and supplies oxygen and nutrients to all of your body's cells. Walking keeps your brain supplied with oxygen.

- Reducing your daily calorie intake by just 20-25% daily can extend your life by 10-15 years

- Walkers live longer and are illness-free longer than their sedentary counterparts anywhere in the world.

- Regular exercise can help to abate the mental and physical effects that stress has on your body.

Here are 12 steps to a longer life are:

1. Decrease salt intake.
2. Maintain normal weight.
3. Decrease cholesterol in the diet.
4. Decrease saturated fat in the diet.
5. Increase the fiber in your diet.
6. Increase consumption of green and yellow vegetables.
7. Avoid the use of smoked-meats and smoked-fishes.
8. Avoid the use of excess caffeine.
9. Avoid the use of tobacco.
10. Avoid excess alcohol consumption.
11. Avoid prolonged exposure to the sun.
12. Avoid stress whenever possible.

Walk as if your life depended on it—It Does!

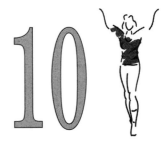

FAT & FIBER COUNTER

INTERPRETING FOOD LABELS

- *Sugar Free*: Less than ½ gram sugar per serving
- *Calorie Free*: No more than 5 calories per serving
- *Salt Free*: Less than 5 milligrams of sodium per serving
- *Low Sodium*: No more than 140 milligrams of sodium per serving
- *Fat Free*: Less than ½ gram fat per serving
- *Low-fat*: No more than 3 grams fat per serving
- *Reduced fat*: At least 25% less fat than comparison food
- *Low Saturated Fat*: No more than 1 gram saturated fat per serving
- *Reduced Saturated Fat*: No more than 50% saturated fat of comparison food
- *Light*: ½ the fat in or ⅓ fewer calories than the regular version of a similar food

SOURCES OF INFORMATION:

- United States Department of Agriculture, Center for Science and Public Interest, Food Manufacturers, Processors and Distributors, *Bowes and Church's Food Values of Portions Commonly Used* (Pennington and Church, 17th Ed.). Scientific Journals and Publications, Author Extrapolations

Bread and Flour

Item	Serving	Tot. Fat (g)	Sat. Fat (g)	Chol. (mg)	Fiber (g)
Bagel, Plain	1 medium	1.1	0.2	0	2
Bagel, Cinnamon Raisin	1 medium	1.2	0.2	0	2
Barley Flour	1 cup	0.5	1.3	0	3
Biscuit					
Plain	1 medium	6.6	1.9	3	1
Buttermilk	1 medium	5.8	0.9	2	1
From Mix	1 medium	4.3	1.2	3	1
Bread					
Cracked Wheat	1 slice	1.0	0.2	0	1
French/Vienna	1 slice	1.0	0.2	0	1
Italian	1 slice	0.5	0.1	0	1
Matzoh	1 piece	0.5	0.1	0	0
Mixed Grain	1 slice	0.9	0.2	0	2
Multigrain, "Lite"	1 slice	0.5	0.0	2	3
Pita, Plain	1 large	0.7	0.1	0	2
Pita, Whole Wheat	1 large	1.2	0.3	0	4
Pumpernickel	1 slice	0.8	0.0	0	2
Raisin	1 slice	1.1	0.3	0	1
Rye	1 slice	0.9	0.2	0	2
Sourdough	1 slice	0.8	0.2	0	1
Wheat, Commercial	1 slice	1.1	0.3	0	2
Wheat, "Lite"	1 slice	0.5	0.1	0	3
White, Commercial	1 slice	1.0	0.2	0	0
White, "Lite"	1 slice	0.5	0.1	0	1
Whole Wheat, Commercial	1 slice	1.2	0.3	0	3
Bread Crumbs	1 cup	1.5	1.3	0	2
Breadsticks	2 small	0.5	0.2	0	0
Bulgar	½ cup	2.0	0.3	0	5.2
Cornbread	1 piece	5.5	2.0	12	1.5
Cornmeal, Dry	½ cup	2.3	0.3	0	6
Cornstarch	1 T	0.0	0.0	0	0
Crackers					
Cheese	5 pieces	4.9	1.6	4	0
Cheese Nips	13 crackers	3.2	1.2	3	0
Cheese w/Peanut Bttr	2 oz. Pkg.	13.5	2.9	7	1
Goldfish, Any Flavor	12 crackers	2.0	0.7	1	0

Item	Serving	Tot. Fat (g)	Sat. Fat (g)	Chol. (mg)	Fiber (g)
Crackers (continued)					
Graham	2 squares	1.3	0.4	0	0
Harvest Wheats	4 crackers	3.6	1.1	0	1
Melba Toast	1 piece	0.2	0.0	0	0
Oyster	15 crackers	2.1	0.3	0	0
Rice Cakes	1 piece	0.2	0.2	0	0
Ritz	3 crackers	3.0	3.0	1	0
Ritz Cheese	3 crackers	3.9	3.9	2	0
Ryekrisp, Plain	2 crackers	0.2	0.2	0	2
Ryekrisp, Sesame	2 crackers	1.4	1.4	0	3
Saltines	2 crackers	0.7	0.7	0	0
Sesame Wafers	3 crackers	3.0	3.0	0	0
Snackwell's Wheat	5 crackers	0.0	0.0	0	1
Sociables	6 crackers	3.0	3.0	0	0
Soda	5 crackers	1.9	1.9	0	0
Tsted w/Peanut Butter	1.5 oz. Pkg.	10.5	10.5	2	0
Triscuit	2 crackers	1.6	1.6	0	1
Vegetable Thins	7 crackers	4.0	4.0	0	0
Wheat Thins	4 crackers	1.5	1.5	0	0
Wheat w/Cheese	1.5 oz. Pkg.	10.9	10.9	1	0
Crepe	1 medium	12.5	12.5	37	0
Croissant	1 medium	11.5	11.5	30	1
Croutons, Commercial	¼ cup	1.8	1.8	0	1
Danish Pastry	1 medium	19.3	19.3	30	1
Doughnut					
Cake	(1) 2 oz.	16.2	16.2	24	1
Yeast	(1) 2 oz.	13.3	13.3	21	1
English Muffin					
Plain	1	1.1	1.1	0	1
w/Raisins	1	1.2	1.2	0	1
Whole Wheat	1	2.0	2.0	0	2
Flour					
Buckwheat	1 cup	3.0	3.0	0	8
Rice	1 cup	1.3	1.3	0	3
Rye	1 cup	2.2	2.2	0	11
Soy	1 cup	16.0	16.0	0	4
White, All Purpose	1 cup	1.2	1.2	0	4
Whole Wheat	1 cup	2.3	2.3	0	12

Bread and Flour (Continued)

Item	Serving	Tot. Fat (g)	Sat. Fat (g)	Chol. (mg)	Fiber (g)
French Toast					
Frzn Variety	1 slice	6.0	6.0	54	0
Hmde	1 slice	10.7	10.7	75	1
Funnel Cake	4 in. diam.	12.8	12.8	48	1
Muffins					
Banana Nut	1 medium	5.0	2.2	20	2
Blueberry, From Mix	1 medium	5.1	1.1	9	1
Bran, Hmde	1 medium	5.8	1.2	16	3
Corn	1 medium	4.8	0.9	18	2
White, Plain	1 medium	5.4	1.1	12	1
Pancakes					
Blueberry, From Mix	3 medium	15.0	4.3	80	4
Buckwheat, From Mix	3 medium	12.3	3.9	75	3
Buttermilk, From Mix	3 medium	10.0	3.2	80	2
"Lite," From Mix	3 medium	2.0	0.6	20	5
Whole Wht, From Mix	3 medium	3.0	1.0	30	6
Phyllo Dough	2 oz.	6.4	0.5	0	1
Pie Crust, Plain	1/8 pie	8.0	1.9	0	0
Popover	1	5.0	2.6	51	0
Rolls					
Crescent	1	5.6	2.8	6	1
Croissant	1 small	6.0	3.5	21	0
French	1	0.4	0.1	0	1
Hamburger	1	3.0	0.8	1	1
Hard	1	1.2	0.3	1	1
Hot Dog	1	2.1	0.5	1	1
Kaiser	1 medium	2.0	0.5	0	0
Raisin	1 large	1.9	0.5	0	1
Rye, Dark	1	1.6	0.1	0	2
Rye, Light, Hard	1	1.0	0.1	0	2
Sandwich	1	3.1	0.4	2	1
Sesame Seed	1	2.1	0.6	1	1
Sourdough	1	1.0	0.0	0	1
Submarine/Hoagie	1 medium	3.0	0.8	3	2
Wheat	1	1.7	0.4	0	1
White, Commercial	1	2.2	1.0	1	0
Whole Wheat	1	1.1	0.2	1	3

Item	Serving	Tot. Fat (g)	Sat. Fat (g)	Chol. (mg)	Fiber (g)
Scone	1	5.5	1.5	28	1
Soft Pretzel	1 medium	1.5	0.7	2	1.5
Stuffing					
Bread, From Mix	½ cup	12.2	6.0	0	0
Cornbread, From Mix	½ cup	4.8	2.5	43	0
Stove Top	½ cup	9.0	5.0	21	0
Sweet Roll, Iced	1 medium	7.9	2.1	20	1
Toaster Pastry	1	5.0	0.8	0	0
Tortilla					
Corn (Unfried)	1 medium	1.1	0.2	0	1
Flour	1 medium	2.5	1.1	0	1
Turnover, Fruit Filled	1	15.0	3.7	0	1
Waffle					
Frozen	1 medium	3.2	0.8	11	1
Hmde	1 medium	9.5	4.1	50	1
From Mix	1 medium	8.5	3.0	48	1

CEREALS

Item	Serving	Tot. Fat (g)	Sat. Fat (g)	Chol. (mg)	Fiber (g)
All Bran	⅓ cup	0.5	0.1	0	10
Apple Jacks	1 cup	0.1	0.0	0	1
Bran, 100%	½ cup	1.9	0.3	0	9
Bran Chex	1 cup	1.2	0.2	0	9
Bran Flakes, 40%	1 cup	0.7	0.1	0	6
Cheerios	1 cup	1.6	0.3	0	2
Cocoa Krispies	1 cup	0.5	0.2	0	0
Corn Chex	1 cup	0.1	0.0	0	1
Cornflakes	1 cup	0.1	0.0	0	1
Cracklin' Oat Bran	⅓ cup	2.7	1.3	0	3
Cream of Wheat w/o Fat	½ cup	0.3	0.0	0	0
Crispix	1 cup	0.0	0.0	0	1
Fiber One	1 cup	2.0	0.4	0	13
Frosted Bran, Kellogg's	¾ cup	0.0	0.0	0	3
Frosted Mini-Wheats	4 biscuits	0.3	0.0	0	1
Fruit and Fiber w/Dates, Raisins					
Walnuts	⅔ cup	2.0	0.3	0	5
w/Peaches, Almonds	⅔ cup	2.0	0.3	0	5

Cereals (continued)

Item	Serving	Tot. Fat (g)	Sat. Fat (g)	Chol. (mg)	Fiber (g)
Fruitful Bran	⅔ cup	0.0	0.0	0	5
Fruit Loops	1 cup	0.5	0.0	0	1
Golden Grahams	¾ cup	1.1	0.1		1
Granola					
Commercial Brands	⅓ cup	4.9	1.8	0	3
Low-Fat, Kellogg's	⅓ cup	2.0	0.0	0	2
Grapenut Flakes	1 cup	0.4	0.2	0	2
Grapenuts	¼ cup	0.1	0.0	0	2
Life, Plain Or Cinn.	1 cup	2.5	0.5	0	4
Mueslix, Kellogg's	½ cup	1.0	0.8	0	5
Nutri-Grain, Kellogg's					
Almond Raisin	⅔ cup	2.0	0.4	0	3
Raisin Bran	1 cup	1.0	0.1	0	5
Wheat	⅔ cup	0.3	0.0	0	3
Oat Bran, Cooked Cereal					
w/o Added Fat	½ cup	0.5	0.1	0	2
Oats					
Instant	1 packet	1.7	0.2	0	1
w/o Added Fat	½ cup	1.2	0.2	0	1
Product 19	1 cup	0.2	0.0	0	1
Puffed Rice	1 cup	0.2	0.0	0	1
Puffed Wheat	1 cup	0.1	0.0	0	1
Raisin Bran	1 cup	0.8	0.1	0	5
Rice Chex	1 cup	0.1	0.0	0	1
Rice Krispies	1 cup	0.2	0.0	0	0
Shredded Wheat	1 cup	0.3	0.0	0	2
Special K	1 cup	0.1	0.0	0	0
Sugar Frosted Flakes	1 cup	0.5	0.1	0	1
Total	1 cup	0.7	0.1	0	2
Total Raisin Bran	1 cup	1.0	0.1	0	5
Wheat Chex	1 cup	1.2	0.2	0	6
Wheaties	1 cup	0.5	0.1	0	2

DAIRY PRODUCTS (CHEESES)

Item	Serving	Tot. Fat (g)	Sat. Fat (g)	Chol. (mg)	Fiber (g)
American					
Processed	1 oz.	8.9	5.6	27	0
Reduced Calorie	1 oz.	2.0	1.0	12	0
Blue	1 oz.	8.2	5.3	21	0
Borden's Fat Free	1 oz.	<0.5	<0.3	<5	0
Borden's Lite Line	1 oz.	2.0	<1.0	NA	0
Caraway	1 oz.	8.3	5.4	30	0
Cheddar	1 oz.	9.2	5.0	26	0
Cheese Sauce	¼ cup	9.8	4.3	20	0
Cheese Spread, Kraft	1 oz.	6.0	3.8	16	0
Cheez Whiz	1 oz.	6.0	3.1	16	0
Cottage Cheese					
1% Fat	½ cup	1.2	0.8	5	0
2% Fat	½ cup	2.2	1.4	10	0
Creamed	½ cup	5.1	3.2	17	0
Cream Cheese					
Kraft Free	1 oz. (2T)	0.0	0.0	5	0
Lite	1 oz. (2T)	6.6	4.2	20	0
Regular	1 oz. (2T)	9.9	6.2	31	0
Edam	1 oz.	7.9	5.0	25	0
Feta	1 oz.	6.0	4.2	25	0
Gouda	1 oz.	7.8	5.0	32	0
Jarlsberg	1 oz.	6.9	4.2	16	0
Kraft American Singles	1 oz.	7.5	4.3	25	0
Kraft Free Singles	1 oz.	0.0	0.0	5	0
Kraft Light Singles	1 oz.	4.0	2.0	15	0
Light N'lively Singles	1 oz.	4.0	2.0	15	0
Monterey Jack	1 oz.	8.6	5.0	30	0
Mozzarella					
Part Skim	1 oz.	4.5	2.4	16	0
Whole Milk	1 oz.	6.1	3.7	22	0
Muenster	1 oz.	8.5	5.4	27	0
Parmesan					
Grated	1 T	1.5	1.0	4	0
Hard	1 oz.	7.3	4.7	19	0
Pimento Cheese Spread	1 oz.	8.9	5.6	27	0

Dairy Products (Cheeses) continued

Item	Serving	Tot. Fat (g)	Sat. Fat (g)	Chol. (mg)	Fiber (g)
Provolone	1 oz.	7.6	4.8	20	0
Ricotta					
"Lite" Reduced Fat	½ cup	4.0	2.4	15	0
Part Skim	½ cup	9.8	6.1	38	0
Whole Milk	½ cup	16.1	10.3	63	0
Romano	1 oz.	7.6	4.9	29	0
Roquefort	1 oz.	7.8	5.0	24	0
Swiss					
Alpine Lace	1 oz.	1.5	0.5	5	0
Sliced	1 oz.	7.8	5.0	26	0
Velveeta	1 oz.	7.0	4.0	20	0
Velveeta Light	1 oz.	4.0	2.0	15	0

Eggs

Item	Serving	Tot. Fat (g)	Sat. Fat (g)	Chol. (mg)	Fiber (g)
Boiled-Poached	1	5.6	1.6	213	0
Fried w/ ½ T Margarine	1 large	7.6	2.7	240	0
Omelet					
2 Oz. Cheese, 3 Egg	1	37.0	12.3	480	0
Plain, 3 Egg	1	21.3	5.2	430	0
Spanish, 2 Egg	1	18.0	5.9	375	1
Scrambled w/Milk	1 large	8.0	2.8	214	0
Substitute, Frzn	¼ cup	0.0	0.0	0	0
White	1 large	0.0	0.0	0	0
Yolk	1 large	5.6	1.6	213	0

MILK AND YOGURT

Item	Serving	Tot. Fat (g)	Sat. Fat (g)	Chol. (mg)	Fiber (g)
Buttermilk					
1% Fat	1 cup	2.2	1.3	9	0
Dry	1 T	0.4	0.2	5	0
Chocolate Milk					
2% Fat	1 cup	5.0	3.1	17	0
Whole	1 cup	8.5	5.3	30	0
Evaporated Milk					
Skim	½ cup	0.4	0.0	0	0
Whole	½ cup	9.5	5.8	37	0
Hot Cocoa					
Mix w/Water	1 cup	3.0	0.7	5	0
w/Skim Milk	1 cup	2.0	0.9	12	0
w/Whole Milk	1 cup	9.1	5.6	33	0
Low-fat Milk					
½% Fat	1 cup	1.0	4.0	10	0
1% Fat	1 cup	2.6	1.6	10	0
2% Fat	1 cup	4.7	2.9	18	0
Milkshake					
Choc. Thick	1 cup	6.1	3.8	24	1
Vanilla, Thick	1 cup	6.9	4.3	27	0
Skim Milk					
Liquid	1 cup	0.4	0.3	4	0
Nonfat Dry Powder	¼ cup	0.2	0.2	6	0
Whole Milk					
3.5% Fat	1 cup	8.2	5.0	34	0
Dry Powder	¼ cup	8.6	5.4	31	0
Yogurt					
Frzn, Low-fat	½ cup	3.0	2.0	10	0
Frzn, Nonfat	½ cup	0.2	0.0	0	0
Fruit Flavored, Low-fat	1 cup	2.6	0.1	10	0
Plain Yogurt					
Low-fat	1 cup	3.5	2.3	14	0
Skim (Nonfat)	1 cup	0.4	0.3	4	0
Whole Milk	1 cup	7.4	4.8	29	0

Desserts

Item	Serving	Tot. Fat (g)	Sat. Fat (g)	Chol. (mg)	Fiber (g)
Apple Betty	½ cup	13.3	2.7	0	3
Baklava	1 piece	29.2	7.2	7	2
Brownie					
Choc., Plain	1	5.0	1.5	14	0
Choc. w/Frosting	1	9.0	1.5	20	1
Choc. w/Nuts	1	7.3	1.8	10	1
Cake					
Angel Food	1/8 cake	0.1	0.0	0	0
Banana	1/8 cake	14.5	2.5	50	1
Black Forest	1/8 cake	15.0	2.0	50	1
Carrot w/Frosting	1/8 cake	18.0	3.6	53	3
Choc. w/Frosting	1/8 cake	16.0	4.0	77	2
Coconut w/Frosting	1/8 cake	17.0	5.4	51	2
Coffee Cake	1/8 cake	6.1	1.0	42	1
Devil's Food, "Light" From Mix	1/8 cake	2.8	1.1	42	0
German Choc. w/ Frosting	1/8 cake	17.0	4.1	72	2
Gingerbread	1/8 cake	2.6	0.9	1.3	0
Lemon Chiffon	1/8 cake	3.0	0.7	3	0
Marble w/Frosting	1/8 cake	15.0	2.5	62	1
Pound	1/8 cake	8.2	4.0	50	1
Spice w/Frosting	1/8 cake	10.2	2.8	48	1
Sponge	1/8 cake	2.0	0.5	50	0
White w/Frosting	1/8 cake	13.1	3.0	30	1
White, "Light", From Mix	1/8 cake	2.6	0.5	15	0
Yellow, "Light", From Mix	1/8 cake	3.0	1.2	35	0
Yellow w/Frosting	1/8 cake	14.0	4.0	50	1
Cheesecake, Traditional	1/8 pie	22.0	10.4	36	0
Cobbler					
w/Biscuit Topping	½ cup	6.0	1.7	2	3
w/Pie-Crust Topping	½ cup	9.3	3.6	5	3
Cookies					
Animal	15 cookies	4.7	1.2	0	0

Item	Serving	Tot. Fat (g)	Sat. Fat (g)	Chol. (mg)	Fiber (g)
Cookies (continued)					
Chantilly, Pepperidge Farm	1	2.0	1.0	<5	0
Choc.	1	3.3	1.0	6	0
Choc. Chip Hmde	1	3.7	2.0	8	0
Choc. Chip, Pepperidge Farm	1	2.5	1.4	<5	0
Choc. Sandwich (Oreo Type)	1	2.1	0.4	0	0
Entenmann's Fat-Free	2	0.0	0.0	0	0
Fat-Free Newtons	1	0.0	0.0	0	0
Fig Bar	1	1.0	0.2	0	1
Fig Newtons	1	1.0	0.3	0	0
Gingersnap	1	1.6	0.3	0	0
Graham Cracker, Choc. Covered	1	3.1	0.9	0	0
Macaroon, Coconut	1	3.4	1.3	0	0
Oatmeal	1	3.2	0.6	0	0
Oatmeal Raisin	1	3.0	0.8	0	0
Peanut Butter	1	3.2	1.0	6	1
Rice Krispie Bar	1	0.9	0.3	0	0
Shortbread	1	2.3	0.4	2	0
Cupcake					
Choc. w/Icing	1	5.5	2.1	22	1
Yellow w/Icing	1	6.0	2.3	23	1
Custard, Baked	½ cup	6.9	3.4	123	0
Date Bar	1 bar	2.0	0.7	2	1
Dumpling, Fruit	1 piece	15.1	5.5	8	2
Éclair (With Choc. Icing & Custard)	1 small	15.4	5.7	115	0
Fruitcake	1 piece	6.2	1.4	11	1
Fruit Ice, Italian	½ cup	0.0	0.0	0	0
Fudgesicle	1 bar	0.4	0.2	3	1
Granola Bar	1 bar	6.8	1.5	0	1
Ice Cream					
Choc. (10% Fat)	½ cup	7.3	4.5	23	1
Choc. (16% Fat)	½ cup	17.0	8.9	44	0
Dietetic, Sugar-Free	½ cup	3.5	1.3	27	0
Vanilla Soft Serve	½ cup	11.3	6.4	76	0

Desserts (Continued)

Item	Serving	Tot. Fat (g)	Sat. Fat (g)	Chol. (mg)	Fiber (g)
Ice Cream (continued)					
Strawberry (10% Fat)	½ cup	6.0	4.0	28	0
Vanilla (10% Fat)	½ cup	7.0	5.4	28	0
Vanilla (16% Fat)	½ cup	11.9	7.4	44	0
Ice Cream Bar					
Choc. Coated	1 bar	11.5	10.0	23	0
Toffee Crunch	1 bar	10.2	7.0	9	1
Ice Cream Cake Roll	1 slice	6.9	4.0	52	0
Ice Cream Cone (Cone Only)	1 medium	0.3	0.1	0	0
Ice Cream Drumstick	1	10.0	4.1	14	1
Ice Cream Sandwich	1	8.3	4.4	12	0
Ice Milk					
Choc.	½ cup	2.0	1.3	9	0
Soft Serve, All Flavors	½ cup	2.3	1.4	7	0
Strawberry	½ cup	2.5	1.2	7	0
Vanilla	½ cup	2.8	1.5	8	0
Jello	½ cup	0.0	0.0	0	0
Ladyfinger	1	2.0	0.5	80	0
Lemon Bars	1 bar	3.2	7.0	13	0
Mousse, Choc.	½ cup	15.5	8.7	124	1
Napoleon	1 piece	5.3	2.6	10	0
Pie					
Apple	1/8 pie	16.9	2.3	3	3
Banana Cream Or Custard	1/8 pie	14.0	10.0	35	1
Blueberry	1/8 pie	17.3	4.0	0	3
Boston Cream Pie	1/8 pie	10.0	3.1	20	1
Cherry	1/8 pie	18.1	5.0	0	2
Choc. Cream	1/8 pie	13.0	4.5	15	3
Coconut Cream Or Custard	1/8 pie	19.0	7.0	80	1
Key Lime	1/8 pie	19.0	6.8	10	1
Lemon Chiffon	1/8 pie	13.5	3.7	15	1
Lemon Meringue, Traditional	1/8 pie	13.1	5.1	50	1
Peach	1/8 pie	17.7	4.6	3	3

Item	Serving	Tot. Fat (g)	Sat. Fat (g)	Chol. (mg)	Fiber (g)
Pie (continued)					
Pecan	1/8 pie	23.0	3.5	100	2
Pumpkin	1/8 pie	16.8	5.7	109	
Raisin	1/8 pie	12.9	3.1	0	1
Rhubarb	1/8 pie	17.1	4.5	2	3
Strawberry	1/8 pie	9.1	4.5	2	1
Sweet Potato	1/8 pie	18.2	6.0	70	2
Pie Tart, Fruit Filled	1	18.7	6.2	23	2
Popsicle	1 bar	0.0	0.0	0	0
Pudding					
Any Flavor Except Choc.	½ cup	4.3	2.5	70	0
Bread w/Raisins	½ cup	7.4	2.9	79	1
Choc. w/Whole Milk	½ cup	5.7	3.1	17	1
From Mix w/Skim Milk	½ cup	0.0	0.0	0	0
Rice w/Whole Milk	½ cup	4.4	2.5	16	1
Sugar Free Varieties	½ cup	2.2	1.4	10	0
Tapioca, w/2% Milk	½ cup	2.4	1.5	8	0
Pudding Pop, Frzn	1 bar	2.0	1.0	2	0
Sherbert	½ cup	1.0	0.5	7	0
Souffle, Choc.	½ cup	3.9	1.4	42	0
Strudel, Fruit	½ cup	1.2	0.1	2	1
Toppings					
Butterscotch/Caramel	3 T	0.1	0.0	0	0
Cherry	3 T	0.1	0.0	0	0
Choc. Fudge	2 T	4.0	2.0	0	0
Choc. Syrup, Hershey	2 T	0.4	0.2	0	0
Marshmallow	3 T	0.0	0.0	0	0
Milk Choc. Fudge	2 T	5.0	2.9	5	0
Pecans In Syrup	3 T	2.8	1.1	0	2
Pineapple	3 T	0.2	0.0	0	0
Strawberry	3 T	0.1	0.0	0	0
Whipped Topping					
Aerosol	¼ cup	3.6	1.4	0	0
From Mix	¼ cup	2.0	1.2	4	0
Frzn, Tub	¼ cup	4.8	3.6	0	0
Non-Fat	1 T	0.0	0.0	0	0

Desserts (continued)

Item	Serving	Tot. Fat (g)	Sat. Fat (g)	Chol. (mg)	Fiber (g)
Whipping Cream					
Heavy, Fluid	1 T	5.6	3.5	21	0
Light, Fluid	1 T	4.6	2.9	17	0
Turnover, Fruit Filled	1	19.3	5.4	2	1
Yogurt, Frozen					
Low-fat	½ cup	1.9	1.2	10	0
Nonfat	½ cup	0.0	0.0	0	0

Candy

Item	Serving	Tot. Fat (g)	Sat. Fat (g)	Chol. (mg)	Fiber (g)
Butterscotch					
Candy	6 pieces	1.3	0.4	0	0
Chips	1 oz.	8.3	6.8	0	0
Candied Fruit					
Apricot	1 oz.	0.1	0.0	0	1
Cherry	1 oz.	0.1	0.0	0	1
Citrus Peel	1 oz.	0.1	0.0	0	1
Figs	1 oz.	0.1	0.0	0	2
Candy Bar (Average)	1 oz.	8.5	4.5	5	1
Caramels					
Plain Or Choc. w/Nuts	1 oz.	4.6	2.2	10	0
Plain Or Choc. w/o Nuts	1 oz.	3.0	1.3	9	0
Choc.-Covered Cherries	1 oz.	4.9	2.9	1	1
Choc.-Covered Cream Center	1 oz.	4.9	2.6	1	1
Choc.-Covered Mint Patty	1 small	1.5	0.8	8	0
Choc.-Covered Peanuts	1 oz.	11.7	4.6	8	2
Choc.-Covered Raisins	1 oz.	4.9	2.9	3	1
Choc. Kisses	6 pieces	9.0	5.0	6	1
Choc. Stars	6 pieces	8.1	4.7	5	12
Cracker Jack	1 cup	3.3	0.4	0	0
English Toffee	1 oz.	2.8	1.7	5	
Fudge					
Choc.	1 oz.	3.4	1.5	1	0
Choc. w/Nuts	1 oz.	4.9	1.2	1	0

Item	Serving	Tot. Fat (g)	Sat. Fat (g)	Chol. (mg)	Fiber (g)
Gumdrops	28 pieces	0.2	0.0	0	0
Gummy Bears	1 oz.	0.1	0.0	0	0
Hard Candy	6 pieces	0.3	0.0	0	0
Jelly Beans	1 oz.	0.0	0.0	0	0
Licorice	1 oz.	0.1	0.0	0	0
Life Savers	5 pieces	0.1	0.0	0	0
M&M's					
Choc. Only	1 oz.	5.6	2.4	3	1
Peanut	1 oz.	7.8	2.4	4	1
Malted-Milk Balls	1 oz.	7.1	4.2	3	1
Marshmallow	1 large	0.0	0.0	0	0
Mints	14 pieces	0.6	0.0	0	0
Peanut Brittle	1 oz.	7.7	1.2	0	1
Peanut Butter Cups	1 oz.	9.2	3.6	3	1
Peppermint Pattie	1 oz.	3.0	2.0	0	<1
Raisinettes	1 oz.	5.5	3.0	4	0
Reese's Pieces	1.7 oz. pkg.	13.0	5.2	2	0
Sour Balls	1 oz.	0.0	0.0	0	0
Taffy	1 oz.	1.5	0.4	0	0
Tootsie Roll Pop	1 oz.	0.6	0.2	0	0
Tootsie Roll	1 oz.	2.3	0.6	0	1

Fats

Item	Serving	Tot. Fat (g)	Sat. Fat (g)	Chol. (mg)	Fiber (g)
Bacon Fat	1 T	14.0	6.4	0	0
Beef, Separable Fat	1 oz.	23.3	6.0	0	0
Butter					
Solid	1 t	3.8	2.4	0	0
Whipped	1 t	2.6	1.6	0	0
Butter Buds, Liquid	2 T	0.0	0.0	0	0
Butter Sprinkles	½ t	0.0	0.0	0	0
Chicken Fat, Raw	1 T	12.8	3.8	0	0
Cream					
Light	1 T	2.9	1.8	0	0
Medium (25% Fat)	1 T	3.8	2.3	0	0
Whipping, Light	1T	4.6	2.9	0	0

Fats (continued)

Item	Serving	Tot. Fat (g)	Sat. Fat (g)	Chol. (mg)	Fiber (g)
Cream, Substitute					
Liquid/Frzn	½ fl. oz.	1.5	1.4	0	0
Powdered	1 T	0.7	0.7	0	0
Half & Half	1 T	1.7	1.1	0	0
Margarine					
Liquid Or Soft Tub	1 t	3.8	0.6	0	0
Reduced Calorie Tub	1 t	2.0	0.3	0	0
Solid (Corn), Stick	1 t	3.8	0.6	0	0
Fat-Free Tub	1 t	0.0	0.0	0	0
Mayonnaise					
Fat-Free	1 T	0.0	0.0	0	0
Reduced Calorie	1 T	5.0	0.7	0	0
Regular	1 T	12.0	1.3	0	0
No-Stick Spray (Pam, etc.)	2-sec spray	0.9	0.2	0	0
Oil					
Canola	1 T	13.6	1.0	0	0
Corn	1 T	13.6	1.7	0	0
Olive	1 T	13.5	1.8	0	0
Safflower	1 T	13.6	1.2	0	0
Soybean	1 T	13.6	2.0	0	0
Pork Fat (Lard)	1 T	12.8	5.0	0	0
Sandwich Spread (Miracle Whip Type)	1 T	4.9	0.7	0	0
Shortening, Vegetable	1 T	12.8	3.2	0	0
Sour Cream					
Cultured	1 T	3.0	1.9	0	0
Fat-Free	1 T	0.0	0.0	0	0
Half & Half, Cultured	1 T	1.8	1.1	0	0
Low-fat	1 T	1.8	1.1	0	0

FISH (ALL BAKED/BROILED W/O ADDED FAT UNLESS OTHERWISE NOTED)

Item	Serving	Tot. Fat (g)	Sat. Fat (g)	Chol. (mg)	Fiber (g)
Abalone, Canned	3 oz.	5.2	0.3	80	0
Anchovy, Canned In Oil	3 fillets	1.2	0.3	10	0
Bass					
Freshwater	3 oz.	4.5	0.9	60	0
Saltwater, Black	3 oz.	1.0	0.2	50	0
Saltwater, Striped	3 oz.	2.3	0.6	70	0
Bluefish					
Cooked	3 oz.	5.2	1.3	50	0
Fried	3 oz.	12.6	2.7	59	0
Butterfish					
Gulf	3 oz.	2.6	0.7	60	0
Northern	3 oz.	10.0	1.9	49	0
Carp	3 oz.	6.0	1.4	72	0
Catfish	3 oz.	3.0	0.7	60	0
Catfish, Breaded & Fried	3 oz.	13.0	2.9	75	1
Caviar, Sturgeon, Granular	1 t	1.5	0.4	47	0
Clams					
Canned, Solids & Liquid	½ cup	0.7	0.1	25	0
Meat Only	5 large	1.0	0.2	42	0
Soft, Raw	4 large	0.8	0.1	29	0
Cod					
Canned	3 oz.	0.6	0.2	45	0
Cooked	3 oz.	0.6	0.2	40	0
Dried, Salted	3 oz.	2.0	0.5	129	0
Crab					
Canned	½ cup	0.9	0.1	60	0
Deviled	3 oz.	10.0	3.5	40	0
Fried, Cake	3 oz.	18.0	4.1	170	0
Crab, Alaska King	3 oz.	1.2	0.2	53	0
Crab Cake	3 oz.	10.6	1.2	100	0
Crayfish, Freshwater	3 oz.	1.2	0.2	115	0
Croaker					
Atlantic	3 oz.	3.0	1.0	60	0
White	3 oz.	0.6	0.3	60	0
Dolphin Fish	3 oz.	0.8	0.2	72	0

Fish (continued)

Item	Serving	Tot. Fat (g)	Sat. Fat (g)	Chol. (mg)	Fiber (g)
Fillets, Frzn					
Batter Dipped	2 pieces	20.0	4.0	40	1
Breaded	2 pieces	18.0	3.0	35	1
Fish Cakes, Frzn, Fried	3 oz.	13.8	3.9	102	2
Flounder/Sole	3 oz.	0.4	0.2	30	0
Gefilte Fish	3 oz.	2.0	0.5	50	1
Grouper	3 oz.	1.2	0.3	45	0
Haddock					
Cooked	3 oz.	0.5	0.1	50	0
Fried	3 oz.	14.0	3.7	60	0
Halibut	3 oz.	1.0	0.5	30	0
Herring					
Canned Or Smoked	3 oz.	16.0	6.0	66	0
Cooked	3 oz.	11.0	2.0	70	0
Kingfish	3 oz.	3.0	0.8	68	0
Lobster					
Broiled With Butter	12 oz.	15.1	8.6	100	0
Steamed	3 oz.	0.5	0.1	70	0
Mackerel					
Atlantic	3 oz.	13.0	1.5	60	0
Pacific	3 oz.	12.5	1.7	55	0
Mussels, Meat Only	3 oz.	2.0	0.7	30	0
Ocean Perch					
Cooked	3 oz.	1.4	0.3	40	0
Fried	3 oz.	11.4	2.8	62	0
Octopus	3 oz.	2.0	0.4	95	0
Oysters					
Canned	3 oz.	2.0	0.8	54	0
Fried	3 oz.	13.7	3.2	83	0
Raw	5 – 8 med	1.8	0.6	54	0
Perch, Freshwater, Yellow	3 oz.	0.8	0.4	80	0
Pike					
Blue	3 oz.	0.7	0.5	75	0
Northern	3 oz.	1.0	0.7	40	0
Walleye	3 oz.	1.0	1.0	80	0
Pompano	3 oz.	9.5	5.0	55	0

Item	Serving	Tot. Fat (g)	Sat. Fat (g)	Chol. (mg)	Fiber (g)
Rainbow Trout					
Baked/Broiled	3 oz.	5.6	1.6	70	0
Breaded, Fried	3 oz.	14.4	3.2	84	1
Red Snapper	3 oz.	1.7	0.5	35	0
Rockfish, Oven Steamed	3 oz.	2.3	0.8	40	0
Roughy, Orange	3 oz.	2.0	0.1	20	0
Salmon					
Atlantic	3 oz.	6.2	0.9	55	0
Broiled/Baked	3 oz.	7.3	2.0	50	0
Chinook, Canned	3 oz.	7.0	2.0	50	0
Pink, Canned	3 oz.	5.0	1.3	54	0
Smoked	3 oz.	9.2	1.0	35	0
Sardines					
Atlantic, In Soy Oil	4 sardines	7.0	0.8	67	0
Skinless & Boneless	3 oz.	6.0	1.5	30	0
Scallops					
Cooked	3 oz.	1.0	0.2	30	0
Frzn, Fried	3 oz.	10.3	2.3	55	0
Steamed	3 oz.	1.2	0.2	40	0
Sea Bass, White	3 oz.	1.3	0.6	40	0
Shrimp					
Canned, Dry Pack	3 oz.	1.4	0.5	155	0
Canned, Wet Pack	3 oz.	0.6	0.3	125	0
Fried	3 oz.	10.5	0.9	120	0
Raw Or Broiled	3 oz.	1.0	0.5	150	0
Sole, Fillet	3 oz.	0.3	0.2	30	0
Squid					
Broiled	3 oz.	1.5	0.5	250	0
Fried	3 oz.	6.4	1.6	275	0
Raw	3 oz.	1.2	0.4	250	0
Sushi Or Sashimi	3 oz.	4.8	1.3	38	0
Swordfish	3 oz.	4.0	1.1	43	0
Trout					
Brook	3 oz.	3.5	0.9	60	0
Rainbow	3 oz.	7.5	1.2	85	0
Tuna					
Albacore	3 oz.	7.3	0.2	70	0
Canned, White In Oil	3 oz.	8.0	1.6	31	0

Fish (continued)

Item	Serving	Tot. Fat (g)	Sat. Fat (g)	Chol. (mg)	Fiber (g)
Tuna (continued)					
Canned, White In Water	3 oz.	1.5	0.5	25	0
Yellowfin	3 oz.	3.0	0.5	57	0
White Perch	3 oz.	3.7	0.7	65	0
Whiting	3 oz.	3.0	0.4	70	0
Yellowtail	3 oz.	5.2	0.9	75	0

Fruit

Item	Serving	Tot. Fat (g)	Sat. Fat (g)	Chol. (mg)	Fiber (g)
Apple					
Dried	½ cup	0.1	0.0	0	5
Whole w/Peel	1 medium	0.4	0.1	0	4
Applesauce, Unsweetened	½ cup	0.1	0.0	0	2
Apricots					
Dried	5 halves	0.2	0.0	0	6
Fresh	3 medium	0.4	0.0	0	2
Avocado					
California	1 (6 oz.)	30.0	4.5	0	4
Florida	1 (11 oz.)	28.0	4.3	0	4
Blackberries					
Fresh	1 cup	0.6	0.0	0	7
Frzn, Unsweetened	1 cup	0.7	0.0	0	7
Blueberries					
Fresh	1 cup	0.6	0.0	0	5
Frzn, Unsweetened	1 cup	0.7	0.2	0	4
Boysenberries, Frzn Unsweetened	1 cup	0.4	0.0	0	6
Cantaloupe	1 cup	0.4	0.0	0	3
Cherries	½ cup	0.8	0.2	0	2
Cranberries, Fresh	1 cup	0.2	0.0	0	4
Cranberry Sauce	½ cup	0.2	0.0	0	1
Dates, Whole, Dried	½ cup	0.4	0.0	0	8
Figs					
Canned	3 figs	0.1	0.0	0	9
Dried, Uncooked	10 figs	1.1	0.4	0	10
Fresh	1 medium	0.2	0.0	0	2

Item	Serving	Tot. Fat (g)	Sat. Fat (g)	Chol. (mg)	Fiber (g)
Fruit Cocktail, Canned w/ Juice	1 cup	0.3	0.0	0	5
Fruit Roll-Up	1	0.0	0.0	0	0
Grapefruit	½ med.	0.1	0.0	0	1
Grapes, Seedless	½ cup	0.1	0.0	0	1
Guava, Fresh	1 medium	0.5	0.2	0	7
Honeydew Melon, Fresh	¼ small	0.1	0.0	0	1
Kiwi, Fresh	1 medium	0.3	0.0	0	2
Kumquat, Fresh	1 medium	0.0	0.0	0	1
Lemon, Fresh	1 medium	0.2	0.0	0	1
Lime, Fresh	1 medium	0.1	0.0	0	1
Mandarin Oranges, Canned w/Juice	½ cup	0.0	0.0	0	4
Mango, Fresh	1 medium	0.6	0.0	0	4
Melon Balls, Frzn	1 cup	0.4	0.0	0	2
Mixed Fruit					
Dried	½ cup	0.5	0.0	0	5
Frzn, Unsweetened	1 cup	0.5	0.2	0	2
Nectarine, Fresh	1 medium	0.6	0.0	0	2
Orange					
Naval, Fresh	1 medium	0.1	0.0	0	4
Valencia, Fresh	1 medium	0.4	0.0	0	4
Papaya, Fresh	1 medium	0.4	0.1	0	3
Peach					
Canned, Water Pack	1 cup	0.1	0.0	0	4
Canned In Heavy Syrup	1 cup	0.1	0.0	0	4
Canned In Light Syrup	1 cup	0.1	0.0	0	4
Fresh	1 medium	0.1	0.0	0	1
Frzn, Sweetened	1 cup	0.3	0.0	0	4
Pear					
Canned In Heavy Syrup	1 cup	0.3	0.0	0	6
Canned In Light Syrup	1 cup	0.1	0.0	0	6
Fresh	1 medium	0.7	0.0	0	5
Persimmon, Fresh	1 medium	0.1	0.0	0	3
Pineapple Pieces					
Canned, Unsweetened	1 cup	0.2	0.0	0	2
Fresh	1 cup	0.7	0.0	0	3
Plantain, Cooked, Sliced	1 cup	0.2	0.0	0	2

Fruit (continued)

Item	Serving	Tot. Fat (g)	Sat. Fat (g)	Chol. (mg)	Fiber (g)
Plum					
Canned In Heavy Syrup	½ cup	0.1	0.0	0	4
Fresh	1 medium	0.4	0.0	0	3
Pomegranate, Fresh	1 medium	0.5	0.0	0	2
Prunes, Dried, Cooked	½ cup	0.2	0.0	0	10
Raisins					
Dark Seedless	½ cup	0.4	0.2	0	6
Golden Seedless	½ cup	0.4	0.2	0	6
Raspberries					
Fresh	1 cup	0.7	0.1	0	5
Frzn, Sweetened	1 cup	0.4	0.0	0	10
Rhubarb, Stewed, Unswetnd	1 cup	0.2	0.0	0	6
Strawberries					
Fresh	1 cup	0.6	0.0	0	3
Frzn, Sweetened	1 cup	0.3	0.0	0	3
Frzn, Unsweetened	1 cup	0.2	0.0	0	3
Tangerine, Fresh	1 medium	0.2	0.0	0	3
Watermelon, Fresh	1 cup	0.5	0.0	0	1

Fruit Juices

Item	Serving	Tot. Fat (g)	Sat. Fat (g)	Chol. (mg)	Fiber (g)
Apple Juice	1 cup	0.3	0.0	0	1
Apricot Nectar	1 cup	0.2	0.0	0	2
Carrot Juice	1 cup	0.4	0.0	0	2
Cranberry Juice Cocktail	1 cup	0.2	0.0	0	2
Cranberry-Apple Juice	1 cup	0.2	0.0	0	1.5
Grape Juice	1 cup	0.2	0.0	0	1
Grapefruit Juice	1 cup	0.2	0.0	0	1.5
Lemon Juice	2 T	0.0	0.0	0	0
Lime Juice	2 T	0.0	0.0	0	0
Orange Juice	1 cup	0.4	0.0	0	1
Peach Juice Or Nectar	1 cup	0.1	0.0	0	1
Pear Juice Or Nectar	1 cup	0.0	0.0	0	1
Pineapple Juice	1 cup	0.2	0.0	0	1
Prune Juice	1 cup	0.1	0.0	0	3
Tomato Juice	1 cup	0.2	0.0	0	2
V8 Juice	1 cup	0.1	0.0	0	2

LUNCH/DINNER COMBOS

Item	Serving	Tot. Fat (g)	Sat. Fat (g)	Chol. (mg)	Fiber (g)
Baked Bean w/Pork	½ cup	1.8	0.8	8	4
Beans					
Refried, Canned	½ cup	1.4	0.5	5	7
Refried, w/Fat	½ cup	13.2	5.2	12	7
Refried, Non-Fat	½ cup	0.0	0.0	0	7
Beans & Franks, Canned	1 cup	16.0	6.0	15	7
Beef & Vegetable Stew	1 cup	10.5	4.9	64	2
Beef Goulash w/Noodles	1 cup	13.9	3.6	87	2
Beef Noodle Casserole	1 cup	19.2	6.5	81	2
Beef Pot Pie	8 oz.	25.0	6.4	40	2
Beef Vegetable Stew	1 cup	10.5	5.0	64	2
Burrito					
Bean w/Cheese	1 large	11.0	5.4	26	4
Bean w/o Cheese	1 large	6.8	3.4	3	4
Beef	1 large	19.0	10.1	70	2
Cabbage Roll w/Beef & Rice	1 medium	6.0	2.7	26	2
Cannelloni, Meat & Cheese	1 piece	29.7	135.0	185	1
Cheese Souffle	1 cup	14.1	5.3	207	0
Chicken A La King, Hmde	1 cup	34.3	12.7	186	1
Chicken A La King w/Rice, Frzn	1 cup	12.0	4.0	122	1
Chicken & Dumplings	1 cup	10.5	2.7	103	1
Chicken & Rice Casserole	1 cup	18.0	5.1	103	1
Chicken & Veg. Stir-Fry	1 cup	6.9	1.2	26	3
Chicken Cacciatore, Frzn	12 oz.	11.0	3.8	80	1
Chicken Fricassee, Hmde	1 cup	18.1	5.2	85	1
Chicken-Fried Steak	4 oz.	23.4	6.8	115	0
Chicken Noodle Casserole	1 cup	10.7	3.2	59	2
Chicken Parmigiana, Hmde	7 oz.	17.0	5.9	150	2
Chicken Pot Pie	8 oz.	25.0	8.4	45	2
Chicken Salad, Regular	½ cup	21.2	9.1	56	0
Chicken Tetrazzini	1 cup	19.6	6.9	50	1
Chicken w/Cashews, Chinese	1 cup	28.6	4.9	60	2
Chili					
w/Beans Only	1 cup	12.0	4.0	35	7
w/Beans & Meat	1 cup	22.4	9.6	110	4

Lunch/Dinner Combos (continued)

Item	Serving	Tot. Fat (g)	Sat. Fat (g)	Chol. (mg)	Fiber (g)
Chop Suey w/Rice Or Noodles	1 cup	10.5	3.6	50	2
Chow Mein, Chicken	1 cup	6.0	2.5	60	2
Corned-Beef Hash	1 cup	24.4	7.5	80	2
Crab Cake	1 small	4.5	0.9	90	0
Creamed Chipped Beef	1 cup	23.0	7.9	44	0
Deviled Crab	½ cup	15.4	4.1	50	1
Deviled Egg	1 large	5.3	1.2	109	0
Egg Foo Yung w/Sauce	1 piece	7.0	1.9	107	1
Eggplant Parmesan, Traditional	1 cup	24.0	8.7	31	3
Egg Roll	2	6.8	2.4	40	1
Enchilada					
Bean, Beef & Cheese	8 oz.	14.1	7.3	38	3
Beef, Frzn	8 oz.	16.0	8.7	40	2
Cheese, Frzn	8 oz.	26.3	14.7	61	3
Chicken, Frzn	8 oz.	16.1	6.4	65	4
Fajitas					
Chicken	1	15.3	3.0	41	4
Beef	1	18.2	6.1	34	3
Fettuccine Alfredo	1 cup	29.7	9.3	73	3
Fish And Chips, Frzn Dinner	6 oz.	14.8	4.3	25	3
Fish Creole	1 cup	5.4	0.9	60	2
Frozen Dinner					
Beef Tips And Noodles	12 oz.	15.1	6.2	75	4
Chopped Sirloin	12 oz.	30.1	14.3	130	5
Fried Chicken	12 oz.	29.6	7.4	110	6
Meat Loaf	12 oz.	23.1	6.4	65	4
Salisbury Steak	12 oz.	27.4	13.5	126	4
Turkey And Dressing	12 oz.	22.6	5.0	74	3
Green Pepper Stuffed w/ Rice & Beef	1 medium	13.5	5.8	52	2
Hamburger Rice Casserole	1 cup	21.0	7.7	57	3
Ham Salad w/Mayo	½ cup	20.2	4.4	54	0
Lasagna					
Cheese	8 oz.	12.0	4.8	22	3
w/Beef & Cheese	1 piece	19.8	10.0	81	2

Item	Serving	Tot. Fat (g)	Sat. Fat (g)	Chol. (mg)	Fiber (g)
Lobster					
Cantonese	1 cup	19.6	5.6	240	0
Newburg	½ cup	24.8	14.7	183	0
Salad	½ cup	7.0	1.5	36	0
Lo Mein, Chinese	1 cup	7.2	1.4	11	1
Macaroni & Cheese	1 cup	16.0	5.0	20	0
Manicotti, Cheese & Tomato	1 piece	11.8	6.0	61	2
Meatball (Reg. Ground Beef)	1 med	5.1	2.0	30	0
Meat Loaf w/Reg. Ground Beef	3 oz.	20.2	8.5	102	0
Moo Goo Gai Pan	1 cup	17.2	3.1	66	1
Moussaka	1 cup	8.9	2.8	98	3
Onion Rings	10 average	17.0	6.0	0	1
Oysters Rockefeller	6 oysters	12.5	4.0	70	1
Pepper Steak	1 cup	11.0	3.2	53	1
Pizza					
Cheese	1 slice	10.1	5.2	40	1
Cheese, French Bread, Frzn	5 oz.	13.0	6.7	37	1
Combination w/Meat	1 slice	17.5	9.0	56	1
Deep Dish, Cheese	1 slice	13.5	6.9	45	1
Pepperoni	1 slice	16.5	8.5	44	1
Tomato Only	1 slice	4.0	2.0	2	1
Pizza Rolls, Frzn	3 pieces	6.9	2.0	10	1
Pork, Sweet & Sour w/Rice	1 cup	7.5	2.0	31	1
Quiche					
Lorraine	1/8 pie	43.5	20.1	218	1
Plain Or Vegetable	1 slice	17.6	8.8	135	1
Ratatouille	½ cup	3.0	0.7	0	2
Ravioli, Canned	1 cup	7.3	3.6	20	3
Ravioli w/Meat & Tomato Sauce	1 piece	3.0	0.9	19	0
Sailsbury Steak w/Gravy	8 oz.	27.3	12.3	126	1
Salmon Patty, Traditional	4 oz.	12.5	4.1	94	1

Lunch/Dinner Combos (continued)

Item	Serving	Tot. Fat (g)	Sat. Fat (g)	Chol. (mg)	Fiber (g)
Sandwiches (on whole wheat bread unless otherwise noted)					
BBQ Beef On Bun	1	16.8	5.8	54	4
BBQ Pork On Bun	1	12.2	3.7	56	4
BLT w/Mayo	1	15.6	4.1	23	4
Bologna & Cheese	1	22.5	9.7	42	4
Chicken w/Mayo And Lettuce	1	14.2	1.8	1191	4
Club w/Mayo	1	20.8	5.4	52	4
Corned Beef On Rye	1	10.8	3.2	34	4
Cream Cheese And Jelly	1	16.0	10.8	38	4
Egg Salad	1	12.5	2.5	228	4
French Dip, Au Jus	1	12.5	4.8	58	4
Grilled Cheese	1	24.0	12.4	56	4
Ham, Cheese & Mayo	1	16.0	7.3	29	4
Ham Salad w/Mayo	1	16.9	4.2	40	4
Peanut Butter & Jelly	1	15.1	2.3	10	5
Reuben	1	33.3	11.8	77	4
Roast Beef & Gravy	1	24.5	5.6	55	4
Roast Beef & Mayo	1	22.6	4.9	60	4
Sloppy Joe On Bun	1	16.8	5.8	54	4
Sub w/Salami & Cheese	1	41.3	17.7	109	4
Tuna Salad	1	17.5	2.9	17	4
Turkey & Mayo	1	18.4	1.9	17	4
Turkey Breast & Mustard	1	5.2	1.2	15	4
Shrimp Creole w/Rice	1 cup	6.1	1.2	123	2
Shrimp Salad	½ cup	9.5	1.6	69	1
Spaghetti					
w/Marinara Sauce	1 cup	2.5	1.0	5	2
w/Meat Sauce	1 cup	16.7	5.0	56	2
w/Red Clam Sauce	1 cup	7.3	1.0	17	2
w/Tomato Sauce	1 cup	1.5	0.4	5	2
w/White Clam Sauce	1 cup	19.5	2.6	49	1
Spaghettios	1 cup	2.0	0.5	8	2
Spinach Souffle	1 cup	14.8	7.1	184	2
Stroganoff					
Beef w/Noodles	1 cup	19.6	7.7	72	2
Beef w/o Noodles	1 cup	26.8	10.6	85	1

Item	Serving	Tot. Fat (g)	Sat. Fat (g)	Chol. (mg)	Fiber (g)
Sushi w/Fish & Vegetables	5 oz.	1.0	0.2	10	1
Taco, Beef	1 med	17.0	8.5	54	2
Tortellini, Meat Or Cheese	1 cup	15.4	5.4	238	1
Tostada w/Refried Beans	1 med	16.3	6.7	20	6
Tuna Noodle Casserole	1 cup	13.3	3.1	38	2
Tuna Salad					
Oil Pack w/Mayo	½ cup	16.3	2.7	20	0
Water Pack w/Mayo	½ cup	10.5	1.6	14	0
Veal Parmigiana	1 cup	22.5	10.1	75	0
Veal Scallopini	1 cup	20.4	7.3	132	2
Welsh Rarebit	1 cup	31.6	17.3	NA	0

MEATS (ALL COOKED W/O ADDED FAT UNLESS OTHERWISE NOTED)

Item	Serving	Tot. Fat (g)	Sat. Fat (g)	Chol. (mg)	Fiber (g)
Round, Eye Of, Lean	3 oz.	4.0	1.5	52	0
Beef, Lean, 5-10% Fat By Weight (Cooked)					
Flank Steak, Fat Trimmed	3 oz.	8.0	2.9	82	0
Hindshank, Lean	3 oz.	9.2	4.0	76	0
Porterhouse Steak, Lean	3 oz.	10.2	5.3	90	0
Rib Steak, Lean	3 oz.	9.2	5.0	80	0
Round Bottom, Lean	3 oz.	9.2	3.4	96	0
Roasted	3 oz.	7.2	2.7	81	0
Rump, Lean, Pot-Roasted	3 oz.	7.0	2.5	60	0
Top, Lean	3 oz.	6.2	2.2	89	0
Sirloin Steak, Lean	3 oz.	8.7	3.6	76	0
Sirloin Tip, Lean Roasted	3 oz.	9.2	3.9	90	0
Tenderloin, Lean, Broiled	3 oz.	11.0	4.2	83	0
Top Sirloin, Lean, Broiled	3 oz.	7.7	3.1	89	0
Beef, Regular 11-17.4% Fat By Weight (Cooked)					
Chuck, Separable Lean	3 oz.	15.0	6.2	105	0
Club Steak, Lean	3 oz.	12.7	6.1	90	0
Cubed Steak	3 oz.	15.2	3.3	85	0
Hamburger					
Extra Lean	3 oz.	13.9	6.3	82	0
Lean	3 oz.	15.7	7.2	78	0
Rib Roast, Lean	3 oz.	15.0	5.5	85	0
Sirloin Tips, Roasted	3 oz.	15.0	3.2	85	0

Meats (continued)

Item	Serving	Tot. Fat (g)	Sat. Fat (g)	Chol. (mg)	Fiber (g)
Beef, Regular 11-17.4% Fat By Weight (Cooked) continued					
T-Bone, Lean Only	4 oz.	10.2	4.2	80	0
Tenderloin, Marbled	3 oz.	15.0	7.0	86	0
Beef, High Fat, 17.4-27.4% Fat By Weight (Cooked)					
Chuck, Ground	3 oz.	23.7	9.6	100	0
Hamburger, Regular	3 oz.	19.6	8.2	87	0
Meatballs	1 oz.	5.5	2.0	30	0
Porterhouse Steak, Lean & Marbled	3 oz.	19.5	8.2	80	0
Rib Steak	3 oz.	14.5	6.0	81	0
Rump, Pot-Roasted	3 oz.	19.5	8.2	80	0
Short Ribs, Lean	3 oz.	19.5	8.2	80	0
Sirloin, Broiled	3 oz.	18.5	7.7	78	0
Sirloin, Ground	3 oz.	26.5	9.3	84	0
T-Bone, Broiled	3 oz.	26.5	10.5	90	0
Beef, Highest Fat, = 27.5& Fat By Weight (Cooked)					
Brisket, Lean & Marbled	3 oz.	30.0	12.0	85	0
Chuck, Stew Meat	3 oz.	30.0	12.0	85	0
Corned, Medium Fat	3 oz.	30.0	14.9	75	0
Ribeye Steak, Marbled	3 oz.	38.6	12.0	90	0
Rib Roast	3 oz.	30.0	18.2	85	0
Short Ribs	3 oz.	31.5	10.5	90	0
Lamb					
Lean	3 oz.	8.0	3.4	100	0
Lean & Marbled	3 oz.	14.3	9.0	97	0
Loin Chop					
Lean	3 oz.	8.0	4.2	80	0
Lean & Marbled	3 oz.	22.3	11.7	58	0
Rib Chop					
Lean	3 oz.	8.0	5.0	50	0
Lean & Marbled	3 oz.	21.0	13.0	70	0
Liver					
Beef, Braised	3 oz.	4.8	1.9	400	0
Calf, Braised	3 oz.	6.8	2.3	450	0
Pork					
Bacon					
Cured, Broiled	1 strip	3.1	1.1	5	0

Item	Serving	Tot. Fat (g)	Sat. Fat (g)	Chol. (mg)	Fiber (g)
Pork (continued)					
Bacon (continued)					
Cured, Raw	1 oz.	16.3	6.0	19	0
Canadian Bacon, Broiled	1 oz.	1.8	0.6	14	0
Ham					
Cured, Canned	3 oz.	5.0	1.5	38	0
Cured, Shank, Lean	3 oz.	6.2	3.0	59	0
Marbled	2 slices	13.8	5.0	60	0
Fresh, Lean	3 oz.	6.3	1.5	40	0
Smoked	3 oz.	7.0	2.7	51	0
Smoked, 95% Lean	3 oz.	5.3	1.8	53	0
Loin Chop					
Lean	1 chop	7.7	3.0	55	0
Lean With Fat	1 chop	22.5	8.8	90	0
Rib Chop, Trimmed	3 oz.	9.8	3.5	81	0
Rib Roast, Trimmed	3 oz.	10.0	3.6	83	0
Sausage					
Brown And Serve	1 oz.	9.4	3.1	24	0
Patty	1	8.4	2.9	22	0
Regular Link	1/2 oz.	4.7	1.6	15	0
Sirloin, Lean, Roasted	3 oz.	10.0	3.6	85	0
Spareribs Roasted	6 med	35.0	11.8	121	0
Tenderloin, Lean, Roast	3 oz.	4.6	1.6	78	0
Top Loin Roast, Trimmed	3 oz.	7.5	2.8	77	0
Processed Meats					
Bacon Substitute (Breakfast Strips)	2 strips	4.8	1.0	0	0
Beef, Chipped	2 slices	1.1	0.4	15	0
Beef Breakfast Strips	2 strips	7.0	2.8	26	0
Beef Jerky	1 oz.	3.6	1.7	30	0
Bologna, Beef/Beef & Pork	2 oz.	16.2	6.9	33	0
Bratwurst					
Pork	2 oz link	22.0	7.9	51	0
Port & Beef	2 oz link	19.5	7.0	44	0
Chicken Roll	2 oz.	2.6	1.6	20	0
Corn Dog	1	20.0	8.4	37	0
Corned Beef, Jellied	1 oz.	2.9	1.0	3	0
Ham, Chopped	1 oz.	2.3	0.8	17	0

MEATS (CONTINUED)

Item	Serving	Tot. Fat (g)	Sat. Fat (g)	Chol. (mg)	Fiber (g)
Hot Dog/Frank					
Beef	1	13.2	8.8	27	0
Beef, Fat-Free	1	0.0	0.0	0	0
Chicken	1	8.8	2.5	45	0
97% Fat-Free Varieties	1	1.6	0.6	22	0
Turkey	1	8.1	2.7	39	0
Turkey, Fat-Free	1	0.0	0.0	0	0
Knockwurst/Knackwurst	2 oz link	18.9	3.2	36	0
Pepperoni	1 oz.	13.0	5.4	25	0
Salami					
Cooked	1 oz.	10.0	6.6	30	0
Dry/Hard	1 oz.	10.0	3.0	16	0
Sausage					
Italian	2 oz link	17.2	6.1	52	0
90% Fat-Free Varieties	2 oz.	4.6	1.6	40	0
Polish	2 oz link	16.2	5.8	40	0
Smoked	2 oz link	20.0	9.2	48	0
Vienna	1 sausage	4.0	1.5	8	0
Turkey Breast, Smoked	2 oz.	1.0	0.3	23	0
Turkey Ham	2 oz.	2.9	1.0	32	0
Turkey Loaf	2 oz.	1.0	0.3	23	0
Turkey Roll, Light Meat	2 oz.	4.1	1.2	24	0
Veal					
Blade					
Lean	3 oz.	8.6	3.5	100	0
Lean With Fat	3 oz.	16.5	7.0	100	0
Breast, Stewed	3 oz.	18.5	8.7	100	0
Chuck, Med. Fat, Braised	3 oz.	12.6	6.0	101	0
Cutlet Breaded	3½ oz.	15.0	NA	NA	0

NUTS AND SEEDS

Item	Serving	Tot. Fat (g)	Sat. Fat (g)	Chol. (mg)	Fiber (g)
Almonds	2 T	9.3	1.0	0	2.5
Brazil Nuts	2 T	11.5	2.3	0	2.5
Cashews, Roasted	2 T	7.8	1.3	0	2
Chestnuts, Fresh	2 T	0.8	0.0	0	4
Hazelnuts (Filberts)	2 T	10.6	1.0	0	2
Macadamia Nuts, Roasted	2 T	12.3	2.0	0	2.5
Mixed Nuts					
w/Peanuts	2 T	10.0	1.5	0	2
w/o Peanuts	2 T	10.1	2.0	0	2
Peanut Butter, Creamy	1 T	8.0	1.5	0	1
Peanut Butter, Chunky	1 T	8.5	2.5	0	2
Peanuts					
Chopped	2 T	8.9	1.0	0	2
Honey Roasted	2 T	8.9	1.5	0	2
In Shell	1 cup	17.0	2.2	0	4
Pecans	2 T	9.1	0.5	0	1
Pine Nuts (Pignolia)	2 T	9.1	1.5	0	2
Pistachios	2 T	7.7	0.8	0	2
Poppy Seeds	2 T	3.8	0.3	0	2
Pumpkin Seeds	2 T	7.9	3.0	0	2
Sesame Nut Mix	2 T	5.1	1.5	0	2
Sesame Seeds	2 T	8.8	1.2	0	2
Sunflower Seeds	2 T	8.9	1.0	0	2
Trail Mix w/Seeds, Nuts, Carob	2 T	5.1	0.9	0	3
Walnuts	2 T	7.7	0.3	0	2.5

Pasta, Noodles and Rice

Item	Serving	Tot. Fat (g)	Sat. Fat (g)	Chol. (mg)	Fiber (g)
Macaroni					
Semolina	1 cup	0.7	0.0	0	1
Whole Wheat	1 cup	2.0	0.4	0	3.5
Noodles					
Alfredo	1 cup	25.1	9.8	73	1
Angel Hair	1 cup	1.5	0.5	0	0
Cellophone, Fried	1 cup	4.2	0.6	0	0
Chow Mein	1 cup	8.0	1.6	0	0
Egg	1 cup	2.4	0.4	50	1
Fettucine, Spinach	1 cup	2.0	0.5	0	2
Manicotti	1 cup	1.0	0.2	0	1
Ramen, All Varieties	1 cup	8.0	5.0	0	1
Rice	1 cup	0.3	0.0	0	1
Romanoff	1 cup	18.0	11.9	95	3
Spaghetti, Whole Wheat	1 cup	1.5	0.5	0	3
Spaghetti, Enriched	1 cup	1.0	0.0	0	1
Rice					
Brown	½ cup	0.6	0.0	0	2
Fried	½ cup	7.2	0.7	0	2
Long Grain & Wild	½ cup	2.1	0.2	0	1
Pilaf	½ cup	7.0	0.6	0	1
Spanish Style	½ cup	2.1	1.0	0	0
White	½ cup	1.2	0.0	0	0

POULTRY

Item	Serving	Tot. Fat (g)	Sat. Fat (g)	Chol. (mg)	Fiber (g)
Chicken					
Breast					
w/Skin, Fried	½ breast	10.7	3.0	87	0
w/o Skin, Fried	½ breast	6.1	1.5	90	0
w/Skin, Roasted	½ breast	7.6	2.9	70	0
w/o Skin, Roasted	½ breast	3.1	1.0	80	0
Leg					
w/Skin, Fried	1 leg	8.7	4.4	99	0
w/Skin, Roasted	1 leg	4.8	4.2	85	0
w/o Skin, Roasted	1 leg	2.5	0.7	41	0
Thigh					
w/Skin, Fried	1 thigh	11.3	2.5	60	0
w/Skin, Roasted	1 thigh	9.6	2.7	58	0
w/o Skin, Roasted	1 thigh	4.5	2.4	45	0
Wing					
w/Skin, Fried	1 wing	9.1	1.9	26	0
w/Skin, Roasted	1 wing	6.6	1.9	29	0
Duck					
w/Skin, Roasted	3 oz.	28.7	9.7	84	0
w/o Skin, Roasted	3 oz.	11.0	4.2	89	0
Turkey Breast					
Barbecued	3 oz.	3.0	1.3	42	0
Honey Roasted	3 oz.	2.6	1.1	38	0
Oven Roasted	3 oz.	3.0	1.3	42	0
Smoked	3 oz.	3.3	1.4	49	0
Turkey Dark Meat					
w/Skin, Roasted	3 oz.	11.3	3.5	89	0
w/o Skin, Roasted	3 oz.	7.0	2.4	75	0
Ground	3 oz.	13.2	4.0	85	0
Ham	3 oz.	5.0	1.7	62	0
Turkey Light Meat					
w/Skin, Roasted	3 oz.	8.2	2.3	76	0
w/o Skin, Roasted	3 oz.	3.2	1.0	55	0
Roll, Light Meat	3 oz.	7.0	2.0	43	0
Sliced w/Gravy, Frzn	3 oz.	3.7	1.2	20	0

Salad Dressings

Item	Serving	Tot. Fat (g)	Sat. Fat (g)	Chol. (mg)	Fiber (g)
Blue Cheese					
Fat-Free	1 T	0.0	0.0	0	0
Low Cal	1 T	1.9	0.2	2	0
Regular	1 T	8.0	1.4	0	0
Buttermilk, From Mix	1 T	5.8	1.0	5	0
Caesar	1 T	7.0	0.9	13	0
French					
Fat-Free	1 T	0.0	0.0	0	0
Low Cal	1 T	0.9	0.1	1	0
Regular	1 T	6.4	0.8	0	0
Garlic, From Mix	1 T	9.2	1.4	0	0
Honey Mustard	1 T	6.6	1.0	0	0
Italian					
Creamy	1 T	5.5	1.6	0	0
Fat-Free	1 T	0.0	0.0	0	0
Low Cal	1 T	1.5	0.1	1	0
Item	Serving	Tot. Fat (g)	Sat. Fat (g)	Chol. (mg)	Fiber (g)
Oil & Vinegar	1 T	7.5	1.5	0	0
Ranch Style	1 T	6.0	0.8	4	0
Russian					
Low Cal	1 T	0.7	0.1	1	0
Regular	1 T	7.8	1.1	0	0
Thousand Island					
Fat-Free	1 T	0.0	0.0	0	0
Low Cal	1 T	1.6	0.2	2	0
Regular	1 T	5.6	0.9	0	0

SAUCES AND GRAVIES

Item	Serving	Tot. Fat (g)	Sat. Fat (g)	Chol. (mg)	Fiber (g)
Barbecue Sauce	1 T	0.3	0.0	0	0
Bearnaise Sauce, Mix	¼ cup	25.6	15.7	71	0
Beef Gravy, Canned	½ cup	2.8	1.3	4	0
Brown Gravy					
From Mix	½ cup	0.9	0.4	1	0
Hmde	¼ cup	14.0	6.5	5	0
Catsup, Tomato	1 T	0.1	0.0	0	0
Chicken Gravy					
Canned	½ cup	6.8	1.7	3	0
From Mix	½ cup	0.9	0.3	1	0
Giblet, Hmde	¼ cup	2.6	0.7	28	0
Chili Sauce	1 T	0.0	0.0	0	0
Cocktail Sauce	¼ cup	0.2	0.0	0	0
Guacamole Dip	1 oz.	4.0	0.7	0	0
Hollandaise Sauce	¼ cup	18.0	10.2	160	0
Home-Style Gravy, From Mix	¼ cup	0.5	0.2	0	0
Horseradish	¼ cup	0.1	0.0	0	0
Jalepeno Dip	1 oz.	1.1	0.4	60	0
Mushroom Gravy					
Canned	½ cup	3.2	0.5	0	1
From Mix	½ cup	0.4	0.2	0	1
Mustard					
Brown	1 T	1.8	0.3	0	1
Yellow	1 T	0.7	0.0	0	0
Onion Dip	2 T	6.0	3.7	13	0
Onion Gravy, From Mix	½ cup	0.4	0.2	0	0
Pesto Sauce	¼ cup	29.0	7.3	18	1
Picante Sauce	½ cup	0.8	0.1	0	2
Pork Gravy, From Mix	½ cup	1.0	0.4	1	0
Sour-Cream Sauce	¼ cup	7.6	4.0	28	0
Soy Sauce	1 T	0.0	0.0	0	0
Soy Sauce, Reduced Sodium	1 T	0.0	0.0	0	0
Spaghetti Sauce					
"Healthy"/"Lite" Varieties	½ cup	1.0	0.0	0	3
Hmde, w/Ground Beef	½ cup	8.3	2.3	23	2
Marinara	½ cup	4.7	0.7	0	3

Sauces and Gravies (continued)

Item	Serving	Tot. Fat (g)	Sat. Fat (g)	Chol. (mg)	Fiber (g)
Spaghetti Sauce (continued)					
Meat Flavor, Jar	½ cup	6.0	1.0	5	2
Mushroom, Jar	½ cup	2.0	0.3	0	2
Oil & Garlic	½ cup	4.5	1.5	5	0
Tomato	½ cup	2.2	0.5	0	0
Spinach Dip (sour-cream & mayo)	2 T	7.1	1.8	10	1
Steak Sauce					
A-1	1 T	0.0	0.0	0	0
Others	1 T	0.0	0.0	0	0
Tabasco Sauce	1 t	0.0	0.0	0	0
Tartar Sauce	1 T	8.2	1.5	0	0
Teriyaki Sauce	1 T	0.0	0.0	0	0
Turkey Gravy					
Canned	½ cup	2.4	0.7	3	0
From Mix	½ cup	0.9	0.3	1	0
Worcestershire Sauce	1 T	0.0	0.0	0	0

Soups

Item	Serving	Tot. Fat (g)	Sat. Fat (g)	Chol. (mg)	Fiber (g)
Asparagus					
Cream of, w/Milk	1 cup	8.2	2.1	10	1
Cream of, w/Water	1 cup	4.1	1.0	5	1
Bean					
w/Bacon	1 cup	5.9	6.0	3	4
w/Ham	1 cup	8.5	2.0	3	3
w/o Meat	1 cup	3.0	1.5	2	5
Beef, Canned					
Broth	1 cup	0.5	0.2	1	0
Chunky	1 cup	5.1	2.6	14	2
Beef Barley	1 cup	1.1	0.5	6	1
Beef Noodle Casserole	1 cup	3.1	1.2	5	1
Black Bean	1 cup	1.5	1.2	0	2
Broccoli, Creamy w/Water	1 cup	2.8	1.0	5	1
Canned Vegetable w/o Meat	1 cup	1.6	0.6	0	1

Item	Serving	Tot. Fat (g)	Sat. Fat (g)	Chol. (mg)	Fiber (g)
Chicken					
Chunky	1 cup	6.6	2.0	30	2
Cream of, w/Milk	1 cup	11.5	4.6	27	0
Cream of, w/Water	1 cup	7.4	2.1	10	0
Chicken & Dumplings	1 cup	5.5	1.3	34	0
Chicken & Stars	1 cup	1.8	0.7	5	1
Chicken & Wild Rice	1 cup	2.3	0.5	7	1
Chicken/Beef Noodle or Veg.	1 cup	3.1	1.2	5	1
Chicken Gumbo	1 cup	1.4	0.3	5	1
Chicken Mushroom	1 cup	9.2	2.4	10	1
Chunky Chicken Noodle	1 cup	5.2	1.1	18	2
Chicken Noodle w/Water	1 cup	2.5	0.7	7	0
Chunky Chicken Vegetable	1 cup	4.8	1.4	17	2
Chicken Veggie w/Water	1 cup	2.8	0.9	10	0
Chicken w/Noodles, Chunky	1 cup	5.0	1.4	19	2
Chunky Chicken w/ Rice	1 cup	3.2	1.0	20	2
Chicken Rice w/Water	1 cup	1.9	0.5	7	1
Clam Chowder					
Manhattan Chunky	1 cup	3.4	2.1	14	1
New England	1 cup	6.6	3.6	7	1
Consomme w/Gelatin	1 cup	0.0	0.0	0	0
Corn Chowder	1 cup	10.5	5.0	22	3.5
Crab	1 cup	1.5	0.4	10	0
Fish Chowder, w/Whole Milk	1 cup	13.5	5.3	37	1
Gazpacho	1 cup	1.5	0.5	0	3
Seafood Gumbo	1 cup	3.9	2.7	40	3
Lentil	1 cup	1.0	0.2	0	3
Lobster Bisque	1 cup	14.0	5.5	35	1
Minestrone					
Chunky	1 cup	2.8	1.5	5	2
w/Water	1 cup	2.5	0.8	3	1
Mushroom, Cream of					
Condensed	1 cup	23.1	10.1	30	1
w/Milk	1 cup	13.6	5.1	20	1
w/Water	1 cup	9.0	2.4	2	1
Mushroom Barley	1 cup	2.3	0.4	0	1
Mushroom w/Beef Stock	1 cup	4.0	1.6	7	1

SOUPS (CONTINUED)

Item	Serving	Tot. Fat (g)	Sat. Fat (g)	Chol. (mg)	Fiber (g)
Onion	1 cup	1.7	0.3	0	1
Onion, French w/Cheese	1 cup	7.5	2.5	15	0
Oyster Stew w/Water	1 cup	3.8	2.5	14	1
Oyster Stew w/Whole Milk	1 cup	17.7	2.5	14	0
Pea					
Split	1 cup	0.6	0.2	1	1
Split w/Ham	1 cup	4.4	1.8	8	1
Potato, Cream of w/Milk	1 cup	7.4	1.2	5	2
Tomato					
w/Milk	1 cup	6.0	2.9	17	1
w/Water	1 cup	1.9	0.4	0	0.5
Tomato Beef w/Noodle	1 cup	4.3	1.6	5	1
Tomato Rice	1 cup	2.7	0.5	2	1
Turkey Noodle	1 cup	2.0	0.6	5	1
Turkey Vegetable	1 cup	3.0	0.9	2	1
Vegetable, Chunky	1 cup	3.7	0.6	0	2
Vegetable w/Beef, Chunky	1 cup	3.0	1.3	8	2
Vegetable w/Beef Broth	1 cup	1.9	0.4	2	1
Vegetarian Vegetable	1 cup	1.2	0.3	0	1
Wonton	1 cup	1.0	<1.0	10	1

VEGETABLES

Item	Serving	Tot. Fat (g)	Sat. Fat (g)	Chol. (mg)	Fiber (g)
Alfalfa Sprouts, Raw	½ cup	0.1	0.0	0	0
Artichoke, Boiled	1 medium	0.2	0.0	0	3
Artichoke Hearts, Boiled	½ cup	0.1	0.0	0	3
Asparagus, Cooked	½ cup	0.3	0.1	0	2
Avocado	½ cup	25.0	4.0	0	3.5
Bamboo Shoots, Raw	½ cup	0.2	0.1	0	2
Beans					
All Types, Cooked w/o Fat	½ cup	0.4	0.2	0	9
Baked, Brown Sugar & Molasses	½ cup	1.5	0.2	0	4
Baked, Vegetarian	½ cup	0.6	0.3	0	5
Baked w/Pork & Tomato Sauce	½ cup	1.3	0.5	8	5

Item	Serving	Tot. Fat (g)	Sat. Fat (g)	Chol. (mg)	Fiber (g)
Beets, Pickled	½ cup	0.1	0.0	0	4
Broccoli					
Cooked	½ cup	0.3	0.0	0	7
Frzn, Chopped, Cooked	½ cup	0.1	0.0	0	2
Frzn In Butter Sauce	½ cup	1.5	1.0	<5	2
Raw	½ cup	0.2	0.0	0	1
Brussel Sprouts, Cooked	½ cup	0.4	0.0	0	2
Butter Beans, Canned	½ cup	0.4	0.0	0	4
Cabbage					
Chinese (Bok Choy)	1 cup	0.2	0.0	0	2
Green, Cooked	½ cup	0.1	0.0	0	2
Carrot					
Cooked	½ cup	0.1	0.0	0	2
Raw	1 large	0.1	0.0	0	2
Cauliflower					
Cooked	1 cup	0.2	0.0	0	3
Raw	1 cup	0.1	0.0	0	4
Celery					
Cooked	½ cup	0.1	0.0	0	1
Raw	1 stalk	0.1	0.0	0	1
Chinese-Style Vegetables, Frzn	½ cup	4.0	0.2	0	3
Chives, Raw, Chopped	1 T	0.0	0.0	0	0
Collard Green, Cooked	½ cup	0.1	0.0	0	2
Corn					
Corn On The Cob	1 medium	1.0	0.1	0	4
Cream Style, Canned	½ cup	0.5	0.1	0	4
Frzn, Cooked	½ cup	0.1	0.0	0	4
Cucumber					
w/Skin	½ medium	0.2	0.0	0	1
w/o Skin, Sliced	½ cup	0.1	0.0	0	0
Eggplant, Cooked	½ cup	0.1	0.0	0	2
Green Beans					
French Style, Cooked	½ cup	0.2	0.0	0	2
Snap, Cooked	½ cup	0.2	0.0	0	2
Italian-Style Vegetables, Frzn	½ cup	5.5	0.2	0	2
Kale, Cooked	½ cup	0.3	0.0	0	2

VEGETABLES (CONTINUED)

Item	Serving	Tot. Fat (g)	Sat. Fat (g)	Chol. (mg)	Fiber (g)
Kidney Beans, Red, Cooked	½ cup	0.5	0.0	0	8
Leeks, Chopped, Raw	½ cup	0.1	0.0	0	1
Lentils, Cooked	½ cup	0.4	0.0	0	8
Lettuce, Leaf	½ cup	0.2	0.0	0	1
Lima Beans, Cooked	½ cup	0.4	0.0	0	5
Mushrooms					
Canned	½ cup	0.2	0.0	0	1
Raw	½ cup	0.2	0.0	0	1
Mustard Greens, Cooked	½ cup	0.2	0.0	0	2
Okra, Cooked	½ cup	0.1	0.0	0	3
Olives					
Black	3 med	4.5	0.5	0	1
Greek	3 med	5.0	0.9	0	1
Green	3 med	2.5	0.2	0	1
Onions					
Canned, French Fried	1 oz.	15.0	6.9	0	0
Chopped, Raw	½ cup	0.1	0.0	0	1
Parsley, Chopped, Raw	¼ cup	0.1	0.0	0	0
Peas, Green, Cooked	½ cup	0.2	0.0	0	4
Pickles	1 medium	0.1	0.0	0	0
Pepper, Bell, Chopped, Raw	½ cup	0.1	0.0	0	2
Pimentos, Canned	1 oz.	0.0	0.0	0	0
Potato					
Baked w/Skin	1 medium	0.2	0.1	0	4
Boiled w/o Skin	½ cup	0.1	0.0	0	2
French Fries	½ cup	6.8	3.0	10	2
Hash Browns	½ cup	10.9	3.4	23	2
Mashed w/Milk	½ cup	5.0	1.5	5	1
Potato Pancakes	1 cake	12.6	3.4	93	1
Scalloped	½ cup	6.0	3.5	12	1
Pumpkin, Canned	½ cup	0.3	0.2	0	4
Radish, Raw	½ cup	0.2	0.0	0	1
Rhubarb, Raw	1 cup	0.2	0.0	0	2
Sauerkraut, Canned	½ cup	0.2	0.0	0	4
Scallions, Raw	½ cup	0.2	0.0	0	4
Soybeans, Mature, Cooked	½ cup	7.7	1.1	0	4

Item	Serving	Tot. Fat (g)	Sat. Fat (g)	Chol. (mg)	Fiber (g)
Spinach					
Cooked	½ cup	0.2	0.1	0	3
Creamed	½ cup	5.1	0.7	1	3
Raw	1 cup	0.2	0.0	0	3
Squash	½ cup	0.2	0.0	0	3
Succotash, Cooked	½ cup	0.8	0.1	0	3
Sweet Potato					
Baked	1 medium	0.2	0.0	0	6
Candied	½ cup	3.4	1.2	8	5
Tempeh (Soybean Product)	½ cup	6.4	0.9	0	1
Tofu (Soybean Curd), Raw	½ cup	5.4	0.8	0	1
Tomato					
Boiled	½ cup	0.5	0.0	0	1
Raw	1 medium	0.4	0.0	0	1
Stewed	½ cup	0.2	0.0	0	1
Turnip Greens, Cooked	½ cup	0.2	0.0	0	2
Wax Beans, Canned	½ cup	0.2	0.0	0	2
Yam, Boiled/Baked	½ cup	0.1	0.0	0	3
Zucchini, Cooked	½ cup	0.1	0.0	0	2

Various Snacks

Item	Serving	Tot. Fat (g)	Sat. Fat (g)	Chol. (mg)	Fiber (g)
Cheese Puffs	1 oz.	10.0	4.8	14	0
Cheese Straws	4 pieces	7.2	6.4	5	1
Chex Snack Mix, Traditional	1 oz.	4.0	0.5	0	1
Corn Chips					
Barbecue	1 oz.	9.0	0.2	0	1
Regular	1 oz.	10.0	1.0	0	1
Cracker Jack	1 oz.	2.2	0.3	0	2
Mix (Cereal & Pretzels)	1 cup	2.5	0.5	0	2
Mix (Raisins & Nuts)	1 cup	25.0	3.5	1.5	4
Peanuts In Shell	1 cup	17.0	2.2	0	4
Popcorn					
Air Popped	1 cup	0.3	0.0	0	1
Caramel	1 cup	4.5	1.2	2	1
Microwave "Lite"	1 cup	1.0	0.0	0	1
Microwave, Plain	1 cup	3.0	0.7	0	1
Microwave, w/Butter	1 cup	4.5	1.8	1	1
Pork Rinds	1 oz.	9.3	3.7	24	0
Potato Chips					
Regular	1 oz.	11.2	2.9	0	1
Baked, Lays	1 oz.	1.5	0.0	0	2
Barbecue Flavor	1 oz.	9.5	2.6	0	1
Light, Pringles	1 oz.	8.0	2.0	0	0
Regular, Pringles	1 oz.	12.0	2.0	0	0
Pretzels (Hard)	1 oz.	1.5	0.5	0	1
Superpretzel® (Soft)	1 med.	1.0	0.0	0	2
Rice Cakes	1	0.0	0.0	0	0
Tortilla Chips					
Doritos	1 oz.	6.6	1.1	0	1
No Oil, Baked	1 oz.	1.5	1.0	0	1
Tostitos	1 oz.	7.8	1.1	0	1

SUBJECT INDEX

W

Y

ABOUT THE AUTHOR

F red A. Stutman, M.D. has done extensive research in the fields of exercise physiology, diet, and nutrition at the U.S. Naval Air Development Center and in his private medical practice. As a medical officer in the U.S. Air Force, Dr. Stutman established one of the first walking programs for cardiac rehabilitation patients. Dr. Stutman is the author of 13 books and numerous medical articles on diet, nutrition, and exercise. Following the publication of *The Doctor's Walking Book,* he became known as "Dr. Walk." Dr. Stutman's books have been featured in national and international newspapers and magazines, including *Prevention, Self, Shape, Cosmopolitan, Family Circle, Ms. Fitness, New Woman, Readers Digest, Star Magazine, The National Enquirer, The New York Times,* and *U.S.A. Today.* Dr. Stutman has appeared frequently on national TV and radio, including *The Today Show* and *Good Morning America.*

Dr. Stutman is currently practicing family medicine as a Temple University Family Practice Physician. He is a Fellow of the American Academy of Family Practice and a recipient of the American Medical Association's Physician's Recognition Award. He is also a member of the American College of Sports Medicine. Dr. Stutman is also the author of the online publication, *Dr. Walk's Diet & Fitness Newsletter.*